ICH - GCP E6(R3) Comprehensive Resource Guide for Clinical Research Professionals

Practical Insights and Key Updates for Clinical Study Design and Application

Alec Spinelli

Copyright Disclaimer

The Book *"ICH - GCP GOOD CLINICAL PRACTICE (GCP) E6(R3) Comprehensive Resource Guide for Clinical Research Professionals – Practical Insights and Key Updates for Clinical Study Design and Application"* is copyrighted. The following disclaimer applies to this publication:

This book is the intellectual property of Alec Spinelli. All rights reserved. No part of this book may be reproduced, distributed, or transmitted in any form or by any means, including photocopying, recording, or other electronic or mechanical methods, without the prior written permission of the publisher, except in the case of brief quotations embodied in critical reviews and specific other noncommercial uses permitted by copyright law. For permission requests, write to the publisher at the address below.

This book is intended for informational purposes only. While every effort has been made to ensure the accuracy and completeness of the information contained within, the author and publisher assume no responsibility for errors, inaccuracies, omissions, or any inconsistency herein. The contents of this book are based on the author's interpretation and research and do not constitute legal, regulatory, or clinical advice. Readers are encouraged to consult official guidelines and relevant regulatory bodies for authoritative information.

Copyright © 2024 by Alec Spinelli. All rights reserved.

Contents

Preface	IV
1. Introduction to ICH GCP E6 R3	1
2. Investigator Responsibilities	13
3. Sponsor Responsibilities	24
4. Ethics and IRB/IEC Responsibilities	35
5. Computerized and Digital Systems	46
6. Monitoring and Auditing	55
7. Data Handling and Record Management	68
8. Risk Management and Quality by Design	80
9. Investigator Brochure	93
10. Clinical Trial Protocol and Protocol Amendments	105
11. Essential Records for the Conduct of a Clinical Trial	118
12. Annex 2 – GCP Considerations for Evolving Clinical Trial Designs	130
13. Conclusion	137
About the Author	142

Preface

As clinical research evolves in response to technological advances, regulatory changes, and emerging challenges, it is more crucial than ever for professionals in the field to have a comprehensive and current understanding of Good Clinical Practice (GCP). Mastering the most recent updates to these standards is vital for conducting successful, ethical, and scientifically sound trials. The ICH-GCP E6(R3) guidelines offer a robust framework that governs the ethical and scientific execution of clinical trials, setting the benchmark for safeguarding the well-being of human subjects and ensuring the accuracy, reliability, and integrity of the data generated from these studies.

This book, titled *ICH - GCP E6(R3) Comprehensive Resource Guide for Clinical Research Professionals – Practical Insights and Key Updates for Clinical Study Design and Application*, is crafted to serve as a critical reference for clinical research professionals at every stage of their careers. Whether you're new to the field or have years of experience, understanding these guidelines is essential for navigating the complex regulatory environment of clinical trials. This book presents a clear and concise exploration of the ICH E6(R3) revision, providing readers with a practical, hands-on approach to applying these updated guidelines in their daily roles.

The ICH-GCP E6(R3) guidelines represent the latest evolution in the ongoing efforts to harmonize the conduct of clinical trials across the globe. These updates reflect the increasing complexity of modern clinical studies and the growing demand for more efficient and risk-based approaches to trial management. The revisions emphasize the importance of flexibility in study design and a proactive approach to risk management, offering a refined set of principles that underscore operational efficiency and regulatory adherence. As a clinical research professional, understanding and integrating these new principles into your workflow is crucial for ensuring the highest quality, ethics, and patient safety standards in the trials you oversee.

For professionals already well-versed in previous GCP guidelines, the E6(R3) updates introduce nuanced changes that are significant and necessary to stay compliant with the shifting regulatory landscape. If you are involved in clinical study design, participant recruitment, monitoring, or data management, this resource will help you grasp the essential updates to GCP and apply them effectively in your daily responsibilities. The comprehensive nature of this guide breaks down the complex and multifaceted aspects of E6(R3) into clear, actionable steps that are easily implemented in the context of clinical trial operations. Whether you are preparing protocols, managing site relationships, or ensuring adherence to ethical standards, this guide will provide you with the tools and knowledge you need to succeed in your role.

One of the central themes of the E6(R3) update is the increased emphasis on risk-based approaches to trial management and monitoring. The new guidelines encourage clinical research professionals to adopt a tailored, flexible approach to study design that focuses on identifying and mitigating potential risks early in the trial process. This proactive strategy ensures that resources are allocated more efficiently and that potential issues are addressed before they escalate into significant problems. In this book, you will explore how to incorporate risk-based management strategies into your study planning, from designing a robust protocol to implementing effective monitoring plans that prioritize critical data points and patient safety.

The E6(R3) revision also strongly focuses on maintaining data integrity throughout the clinical trial process. In an age where technology is increasingly central in data collection, management, and analysis, ensuring that clinical trial data remains accurate, complete, and secure is paramount. This guide will walk you through the best practices for safeguarding data integrity, including tips for handling deviations, maintaining meticulous records, and implementing systems that minimize the risk of data breaches or inaccuracies. You will also learn how to apply these principles in real-world scenarios, ensuring that the data you generate is reliable and compliant with global regulatory standards.

Ethical considerations remain at the heart of the ICH-GCP guidelines, and E6(R3) builds upon this foundation by reinforcing the importance of protecting human subjects throughout the clinical trial process. This guide provides practical insights into how the updated guidelines impact participant safety and outlines strategies for ensuring that ethical standards are maintained at every trial phase. From obtaining informed consent to managing adverse events, this resource offers clear guidance on the ethical challenges you may face in clinical research and how to address them with professionalism and care.

As the landscape of clinical research continues to shift and grow, the roles and responsibilities of clinical research professionals are also evolving. The

E6(R3) updates introduce new expectations for organizing study teams and sharing responsibilities across stakeholders. Whether working in a sponsor or CRO capacity or directly at a clinical trial site, understanding how these updates affect your role is critical for staying ahead in this fast-paced environment. This guide will help you navigate the evolving expectations for clinical research roles, from principal investigators to clinical research associates, ensuring that you remain compliant and practical in your position.

If you are preparing to step into a new role or are seeking to expand your knowledge base, this book is a go-to resource for mastering the fundamental components of the updated GCP guidelines. The clinical research industry is highly competitive, and staying up-to-date with the latest regulatory changes can give you a significant edge in your career. By familiarizing yourself with the E6(R3) guidelines, you position yourself as a knowledgeable, forward-thinking professional equipped to handle modern clinical research demands. This resource will empower you with the insights and tools to navigate the increasingly complex regulatory landscape, ensuring your success in a rapidly changing industry.

In writing this book, my aim is to provide a comprehensive yet accessible resource that helps demystify the complexities of GCP compliance. The information presented in this guide is designed to be immediately applicable to your work, offering practical tips and strategies that you can use to improve your efficiency and effectiveness in managing clinical trials. Whether you are designing a new study, overseeing participant recruitment, or managing trial data, the insights provided in this book will help you navigate the challenges of clinical research with greater confidence and ease.

The importance of staying informed and prepared cannot be overstated in an industry as dynamic and ever-changing as clinical research. Regulatory guidelines are constantly being updated to reflect new developments in science, technology, and ethics, and staying on top of these changes is essential for anyone seeking to advance in their career. This book is not just a reference for understanding the E6(R3) guidelines. It is a tool for your professional development, offering valuable knowledge to help you stay ahead of the curve as the industry continues to innovate and evolve.

The *ICH - GCP E6(R3) Comprehensive Resource Guide for Clinical Research Professionals* is an instrument for understanding the latest updates to Good Clinical Practice. Whether you're a seasoned professional or new to the field, this guide provides the knowledge and strategies needed to navigate the complex regulatory environment of clinical trials. From risk-based study design to data integrity and participant safety, this book covers all the essential elements of E6(R3). It offers practical, actionable insights you can apply directly to your work. As clinical research expands and innovates, staying informed and prepared is paramount to advancing your career and ensuring the success of the trials you oversee.

I hope *the ICH—GCP E6(R3) Comprehensive Resource Guide for Clinical Research Professionals* will be an invaluable resource for your professional journey and a tool you can return to as you continue to navigate the evolving world of clinical research. If this guide provided you with valuable insights, please consider leaving a review on Amazon. Your feedback helps others discover and trust this essential resource and supports clinical research professionals worldwide in finding accurate, reliable guidance. Thank you!

Alec Spinelli

Chapter One

Introduction to ICH GCP E6 R3

1.1 What is ICH GCP?

Good Clinical Practice (GCP) represents an international quality standard for conducting clinical trials involving human subjects, ensuring that ethical and scientific principles guide every aspect of the research. Developed by the International Council for Harmonisation of Technical Requirements for Pharmaceuticals for Human Use (ICH), GCP encompasses a comprehensive framework that governs the planning, execution, documentation, and reporting of clinical trials. Its core objective is twofold: to protect the rights, safety, and welfare of clinical trial participants and to ensure that the data generated during the trials is accurate, reliable, and credible.

The concept of GCP emerged from a necessity to harmonize the diverse regulatory frameworks that govern clinical trials across different regions, including Europe, the United States, and Japan. Before introducing these standards, the inconsistencies across borders posed significant challenges to multinational clinical research, leading to inefficiencies, redundancies, and delays. By establishing a uniform set of principles, ICH GCP facilitates the conduct of clinical trials in a way that satisfies regulatory expectations worldwide, creating a common language for all stakeholders involved in the clinical research process.

At its core, GCP is designed to promote the ethical treatment of participants. Clinical trials inherently involve a degree of uncertainty, with patients often exposed to investigational drugs or therapies that may not have fully understood the risks. To address this, GCP mandates that investigators obtain informed consent from participants, ensuring they are fully aware of the trial's objectives, procedures, potential benefits, and risks. Informed consent must be voluntary, and participants should be free to withdraw from the study without repercussion. This protection of participant rights forms the ethical foundation upon which GCP is built.

Additionally, GCP ensures that clinical trials adhere to scientific rigor. It requires that trials be based on sound protocols developed with the input of qualified experts and follow stringent data collection, analysis, and reporting procedures. Through these measures, GCP ensures that the results of clinical trials are not only ethically conducted but also scientifically valid. This is critical for regulatory agencies when reviewing trial data for the approval of new drugs or therapies, as the credibility of the research directly influences the ability to make informed decisions about the safety and efficacy of new medical products.

For clinical research professionals, understanding and adhering to GCP principles is not just a regulatory obligation but an essential component of professional practice. Investigators, sponsors, and clinical research teams must work in concert to ensure that every aspect of the trial adheres to

GCP standards, from patient recruitment and informed consent to data handling and final reporting. Failure to comply with these standards can result in serious consequences, including regulatory sanctions, trial delays, and reputational damage. Furthermore, non-compliance can undermine the scientific integrity of the research, potentially putting patient safety at risk and compromising the validity of the data collected.

ICH GCP serves as a cornerstone of clinical research, ensuring that trials are conducted in a manner that respects the rights of participants while maintaining the highest standards of scientific integrity. The guidelines provide a robust framework for all clinical trials involving human subjects, regardless of the study's therapeutic area or geographic location. By adhering to GCP, clinical research professionals help foster a climate of ethical responsibility and scientific excellence that ultimately contributes to advancing medical knowledge and developing safer, more effective therapies.

1.2 The Evolution of GCP

The development of Good Clinical Practice (GCP) has been a continuous process shaped by the growing complexity of clinical research and the evolving regulatory landscape. The principles that underpin GCP have remained consistent. Namely, the protection of human subjects and the assurance of data integrity and how these principles are implemented have adapted to keep pace with technological advancements and changes in trial design. The current version, ICH GCP E6(R3), reflects the most recent iteration of these guidelines and builds upon earlier versions to address the modern realities of clinical research.

The origins of GCP can be traced back to various international agreements and declarations established to promote the ethical treatment of human subjects in research. One of the earliest and most influential was the Declaration of Helsinki, adopted by the World Medical Association in 1964. This document laid the ethical groundwork for human subject research, emphasizing the importance of informed consent and the need for independent ethical review. While not legally binding, the Declaration of Helsinki set the stage for developing more formalized guidelines like GCP.

The first formal version of ICH GCP, E6(R1), was introduced in 1996. The global clinical research environment was rapidly expanding at that time, with pharmaceutical companies conducting trials in multiple countries and regions. This posed significant challenges, as each country had its regulatory requirements for clinical trials, leading to a lack of uniformity and efficiency. ICH GCP E6(R1) was developed to harmonize these diverse regulatory frameworks, providing a unified standard for clinical trials across Europe, the United States, and Japan.

E6(R1) provided a comprehensive set of guidelines covering all aspects of clinical trial conduct, from the responsibilities of investigators and sponsors to the ethical treatment of participants and the data collection and reporting requirements. These guidelines quickly became the global standard for clinical research and were widely adopted by regulatory authorities and industry stakeholders. However, as the field of clinical research continued to evolve, it became clear that updates to the guidelines were needed to address emerging challenges.

ICH GCP E6(R2) was introduced in 2016 in response to these changing dynamics. This revision built on the foundations of E6(R1) while addressing several key areas that have become increasingly relevant in modern clinical research. One of the most significant updates in E6(R2) was the introduction of risk-based monitoring (RBM), which provided a more flexible approach to trial oversight. Rather than applying the same level of monitoring to all aspects of a trial, RBM allowed sponsors to focus their resources on the areas that posed the most significant risk to participant safety and data integrity. This shift was significant as trials became more complex, often involving multiple sites and diverse populations.

E6(R2) also recognized the growing role of technology in clinical research. With the widespread adoption of electronic data capture (EDC) systems and other digital tools, the guidelines were updated to reflect the need for robust data management and security practices. E6(R2) emphasized the importance of data integrity in the digital age, ensuring that electronic records and systems meet the same high standards as traditional paper-based methods.

The latest version, ICH GCP E6(R3), takes these updates even further, reflecting the continued evolution of clinical research in the 21st century. One of the most significant changes in E6(R3) is the emphasis on Quality by Design (QbD), a proactive approach to trial planning that focuses on identifying and mitigating risks before they can impact the trial. QbD encourages sponsors and investigators to prioritize the elements of a trial most critical to participant safety and data quality rather than applying a one-size-fits-all approach to trial oversight. This allows for more efficient use of resources and helps ensure that trials are conducted with the highest possible quality standards.

E6(R3) also recognizes the growing trend toward decentralized clinical trials (DCTs), in which participants may be monitored remotely using digital tools and technologies. These types of trials offer significant advantages, particularly regarding participant convenience and recruitment. However, they also present unique challenges in maintaining oversight and ensuring data quality. E6(R3) provides guidance on conducting decentralized trials in a way that maintains compliance with GCP principles, ensuring that the rights and safety of participants are protected regardless of where the trial is conducted.

E6(R3) also emphasizes the importance of patient-centric trial designs. Recognizing that participant engagement is critical to the success of clinical trials, the new guidelines encourage sponsors to involve patients in the trial planning process. This can include seeking input from patient advocacy groups, simplifying trial procedures to reduce participant burden, and offering flexible options for trial participation. By incorporating the patient perspective into trial design, E6(R3) helps ensure that trials are more inclusive and accessible, ultimately leading to better recruitment and retention rates.

The evolution of GCP reflects the broader changes taking place in clinical research. As trials become more complex and technology continues to transform the way research is conducted, the guidelines must adapt to ensure that the core principles of ethics and scientific integrity are upheld. E6(R3) represents the latest step in this ongoing process, providing a flexible and robust framework for the conduct of clinical trials in the modern era.

1.3 Scope and Application

The scope of ICH GCP E6(R3) is comprehensive, covering every stage of the clinical trial process from planning and initiation to data collection, analysis, and final reporting. These guidelines apply to all clinical trials involving human subjects, regardless of the therapeutic area, phase of development, or geographic location. While ICH GCP was initially developed to harmonize pharmaceutical regulations across Europe, the United States, and Japan, it has since been adopted by numerous other regions, making it the global standard for clinical research.

At its core, ICH GCP serves two primary purposes: ensuring the protection of human subjects and ensuring the generation of reliable, credible data. These twin objectives are reflected in every aspect of the guidelines, which provide detailed instructions on the roles and responsibilities of investigators, sponsors, ethics committees, and regulatory authorities. By adhering to GCP, clinical research professionals can ensure that their trials are conducted in a way that meets the highest ethical and scientific standards while complying with their respective regions' regulatory requirements.

One of the fundamental aspects of GCP is its focus on the ethical treatment of participants. Before a trial can begin, it must undergo review and approval by an Institutional Review Board (IRB) or Independent Ethics Committee (IEC). These bodies are responsible for evaluating the proposed trial's scientific validity and ethical soundness, ensuring that the risks to participants are minimized and the potential benefits outweigh the risks. Informed consent is a critical component of this process. GCP requires that all participants be provided with clear, comprehensive information about the trial, including its objectives, procedures, potential risks, and benefits. This ensures that participants can make an informed decision about whether or not to participate in the study.

GCP also emphasizes the importance of scientific integrity in clinical research. The guidelines provide detailed instructions on the development of trial protocols, the collection and analysis of data, and the reporting of results. Investigators must follow the trial protocol strictly, making any necessary amendments only with the sponsor's and ethics committee's approval. Data must be collected to ensure accuracy, completeness, and reliability, with stringent requirements for source data verification and the use of case report forms (CRFs). These measures are designed to ensure that the data generated during the trial is of the highest quality, providing a solid foundation for regulatory decisions.

Another essential aspect of GCP is its flexibility. The guidelines are designed to be adaptable to a wide range of clinical trial scenarios, from small pilot studies to large multinational Phase III trials. This flexibility is crucial in modern clinical research, where trial designs are becoming increasingly complex and innovative. For example, decentralized clinical trials, which allow participants to be monitored remotely using digital tools, have become more common in recent years. E6(R3) provides specific guidance on conducting these types of trials while maintaining compliance with GCP principles, ensuring that the rights and safety of participants are protected regardless of where the trial is conducted.

GCP has broad applicability across different types of trials and is relevant to a wide range of therapeutic areas and phases of development. Whether a trial is investigating a new pharmaceutical product, a medical device, or a biologic, the principles of GCP can be applied to ensure that the trial is conducted in a way that meets the highest ethical and scientific standards. This is particularly important for sponsors seeking regulatory approval for their products, as compliance with GCP is a critical requirement for submission to regulatory authorities.

The global nature of GCP makes it an essential tool for conducting multinational trials. GCP facilitates the conduct of clinical trials across borders by providing a common set of standards recognized by regulatory authorities in multiple regions. This is particularly important for sponsors looking to bring new therapies to market globally, as it allows them to conduct a single trial that meets the regulatory requirements of multiple regions. By adhering to GCP, sponsors can ensure that their trials are conducted in a way that satisfies regulatory expectations while protecting participants' rights and safety.

1.4 Core Principles of ICH GCP

The core principles of ICH Good Clinical Practice (GCP) provide the ethical and scientific foundation for conducting clinical trials that prioritize participant safety, data integrity, and regulatory compliance. These principles serve as a blueprint to ensure trials are ethically conducted, scientifically valid, and aligned with international standards, benefiting both participants and the broader medical community.

One of the primary principles is the emphasis on ethical conduct. Clinical trials must always safeguard participants' rights, safety, and well-being, adhering to guidelines like the Declaration of Helsinki. This commitment is supported by thorough informed consent procedures, which ensure that participants are fully aware of the trial's purpose, risks, and benefits and are free to withdraw at any time without penalty. Scientific soundness is equally vital: trials must be based on robust scientific rationale and previous research, and protocols must be well-structured, with clear objectives, methodologies, and endpoints to generate reliable results.

Qualified personnel must oversee every aspect of the trial. All team members, from investigators to site staff, should be trained and credentialed to conduct trials responsibly. Another cornerstone is data integrity and quality control, which involves accurate, verifiable data collection and rigorous monitoring to maintain data quality and regulatory compliance. Clear and comprehensive documentation ensures reproducibility and consistency across trial sites, allowing accurate assessment and potential replication of study findings.

Compliance with regulatory standards is essential, ensuring that trials meet local and international legal requirements. Adherence to GCP principles facilitates trust and approval from regulatory authorities, contributing to advancing medical knowledge and developing new treatments that can safely and effectively serve public health needs.

1.5 Key Stakeholders in ICH GCP Compliance

The integrity of clinical trials and adherence to ICH Good Clinical Practice (GCP) standards rely on the coordinated efforts of multiple vital stakeholders: sponsors, investigators, Institutional Review Boards (IRBs), and regulatory authorities. Each plays a crucial role in maintaining ethical standards, participant safety, and data reliability.

Sponsors are often pharmaceutical companies, biotechnology firms, or other organizations responsible for funding and overseeing clinical trials. They are tasked with designing scientifically sound protocols, providing investigational products, and ensuring that trials comply with GCP and regulatory guidelines. Sponsors also select qualified investigators and monitor the study's conduct to ensure data accuracy and participant protection.

Investigators are the individuals, often physicians, responsible for conducting the trial at clinical sites. They ensure that the trial is conducted per the approved protocol, that participants provide informed consent, and that accurate data is recorded and reported. Investigators are also accountable for participant safety, monitoring adverse events, and complying with ethical and regulatory requirements.

Institutional Review Boards (IRBs) are independent ethics committees to protect participants' rights and well-being. Before a trial begins, the IRB reviews the protocol to ensure that it is ethically sound and that participant risks are minimized. They continue monitoring the trial's progress, reviewing protocol amendments and safety updates.

Regulatory Authorities, such as the FDA in the United States or the EMA in Europe, are government bodies that oversee trial compliance with legal and ethical standards. They review protocols, approve trials, and inspect sites to uphold GCP principles. By enforcing these standards, regulatory authorities help ensure that trial data is credible and that the investigational product's benefits and risks are accurately assessed.

Together, these stakeholders create a system of checks and balances that upholds the ethical and scientific standards essential to GCP, fostering public trust in clinical research.

The scope and application of ICH GCP E6(R3) are vast, encompassing every aspect of the clinical trial process and ensuring that trials are conducted with the highest ethical and scientific standards. These guidelines provide a flexible, robust framework that can be adapted to a wide range of trial scenarios, therapeutic areas, and phases of development. By adhering to GCP, clinical research professionals can ensure that their trials are compliant with regulatory requirements and conducted in a way that prioritizes the rights, safety, and well-being of participants while generating credible, reliable data for regulatory approval.

This comprehensive introduction to ICH GCP E6(R3) sets the stage for a deeper exploration of the roles, responsibilities, and practices that will be covered in subsequent chapters. Each section of this guide will provide detailed insights into the practical application of GCP, helping clinical research professionals navigate the complexities of modern clinical trials while upholding the highest standards of ethics and scientific rigor.

Chapter Two

Investigator Responsibilities

2.1 Qualifications and Oversight

One of the fundamental pillars of Good Clinical Practice (GCP) is ensuring that individuals conducting clinical trials, particularly investigators, possess the appropriate qualifications, skills, and experience to conduct the study ethically, safely, and effectively. The role of the investigator is pivotal, as they are responsible for overseeing every aspect of the clinical trial at their site, including subject safety, protocol adherence, and the quality of data collected. The integrity of a clinical trial relies heavily on the investigator's competence, attention to detail, and ethical commitment.

Investigators must have the necessary educational background, training, and practical experience relevant to the clinical trial they are conducting. This includes thoroughly understanding the therapeutic area under investigation and knowledge of clinical research principles and regulations. Many countries, in line with GCP guidelines, mandate that investigators hold medical degrees, though other health-related qualifications may be acceptable depending on the nature of the trial. For instance, in non-drug trials, investigators might include professionals such as nurses, psychologists, or other specialists with relevant expertise.

However, qualifications are not limited to formal education. Investigators must also demonstrate a proven track record of conducting clinical research and managing trials of similar complexity. This is crucial because clinical trials involve multifaceted tasks, such as overseeing the enrollment of subjects, maintaining regulatory compliance, and ensuring the integrity of the trial's data. An investigator who is unfamiliar with these responsibilities can jeopardize the study by introducing risks to participant safety or compromising data quality. Regulatory bodies and sponsors often require training specific to the protocol, therapeutic area, and ethical guidelines like GCP to ensure that investigators are adequately prepared.

Oversight is another critical responsibility of the investigator. Once qualified, the investigator must ensure that all aspects of the trial are conducted per the approved protocol, applicable regulations, and GCP guidelines. Effective oversight requires continuous engagement with the trial team, regular monitoring of participant progress, and vigilance in identifying potential issues that could affect subject safety or data quality. Investigators are responsible for delegating tasks appropriately, ensuring that all staff involved in the trial are adequately trained and qualified for their roles. However, while investigators can delegate specific tasks, they cannot delegate their overall responsibility for the conduct of the trial. This distinction is essential because ultimate accountability lies with the investigator.

Good oversight also involves regular communication with the sponsor, ethics committee, and regulatory authorities. Investigators must ensure that they are aware of any amendments to the protocol or changes to the investigational product's safety profile. Prompt reporting of serious adverse events, protocol deviations, and any unforeseen circumstances that could impact the study is an essential aspect of an investigator's oversight responsibilities. Effective communication ensures that all stakeholders are informed of the trial's progress and that any necessary actions are taken to maintain the study's integrity.

An investigator's qualifications and oversight capabilities form the foundation of a successful clinical trial. The investigator's role is to lead the trial at the site level and ensure that it is conducted with the highest ethical standards, safeguarding both the participants' safety and the data's scientific validity. Without qualified and vigilant investigators, the entire trial could be compromised, potentially affecting patient safety and the trial's outcome.

2.2 Ensuring Subject Protection

A core responsibility of the investigator is the protection of human subjects involved in clinical trials. Ensuring subject safety and well-being is a regulatory obligation and an ethical imperative at the heart of Good Clinical Practice (GCP). Investigators must safeguard participants' rights, dignity, and health throughout the trial, from recruitment and informed consent to the management of any risks that may arise during the study.

One of the primary mechanisms for ensuring subject protection is obtaining informed consent. Informed consent is not merely a legal formality; it is a process that involves providing potential participants with all relevant information about the trial, including its purpose, procedures, risks, and benefits, so that they can make a voluntary and informed decision about whether to participate. Investigators must ensure that this information is presented in clear, non-technical language that the participant can easily understand. The process should allow ample time for participants to ask questions and consider their options before agreeing to enroll in the trial. Furthermore, consent must be documented appropriately, with a signed informed consent form retained for the trial records.

The informed consent process is an ongoing responsibility. Throughout the trial, investigators must ensure that participants remain fully informed, particularly if new information that could impact their decision to continue is available. For instance, if new risks are identified or the investigational product's safety profile changes, the investigator must update participants and allow them to re-consent their participation. Investigators must also respect participants' rights to withdraw from the study at any time without coercion or negative consequences.

Risk management is another critical component of subject protection. Clinical trials inherently involve some risk, particularly in early-phase studies where the investigational product's safety and efficacy are not fully established. Investigators are responsible for identifying, assessing, and mitigating risks to participants. This includes ensuring that all trial procedures are performed in accordance with the protocol, which is designed to minimize risk while obtaining scientifically valid results. Investigators must be vigilant in monitoring participants for any signs of anticipated and unanticipated adverse events. Serious adverse events (SAEs), in particular, must be reported to the sponsor and regulatory authorities in a timely manner, as these events may have significant implications for participant safety and the continuation of the trial.

Investigators must also protect participants from undue harm through protocol compliance. The trial protocol is a detailed document that outlines the study's objectives, design, methodology, and procedures. It is developed to ensure that the study is conducted in a scientifically rigorous and ethically sound manner. Investigators are responsible for adhering to the protocol and ensuring that any deviations are minimized, documented, and reported appropriately if they occur. Protocol deviations can occur for various reasons, including logistical challenges or participant non-compliance. However, deviations impacting participant safety or data integrity must be handled carefully.

Investigators are also responsible for ensuring that participants receive appropriate care during and after the trial. This includes providing medical treatment for any adverse events that occur during the study and ensuring that participants have access to any necessary follow-up care once their participation in the trial has ended. Investigators must also be prepared to make difficult decisions about whether to continue, modify, or halt the trial if serious safety concerns arise.

Ensuring subject protection is one of the investigator's fundamental responsibilities in clinical research. From the informed consent process to ongoing risk management and protocol compliance, investigators must prioritize participants' safety and well-being at every trial stage. By doing so, they not only uphold the ethical principles of GCP but also contribute to the scientific credibility of the trial.

2.3 Investigational Product Management

The management of investigational products (IPs) is a critical responsibility for investigators in clinical trials. Investigational products, which include drugs, devices, or other therapies being tested for safety and efficacy, must be handled with the utmost care to ensure participant safety and the integrity of the trial data. Proper management of these products encompasses a range of activities, from accountability and storage to administration and documentation.

The accountability of investigational products is essential to ensure that they are used appropriately and follow the trial protocol. Investigators must maintain accurate records of the receipt, storage, dispensing, and return or disposal of the IP. These records are often referred to as drug accountability logs or device accountability forms, depending on the nature of the investigational product. Accurate accountability records are crucial for several reasons. First, they ensure that the correct dose or amount of the IP is administered to each participant at the appropriate time, reducing the risk of dosing errors. Second, they provide a traceable record of the IP's use, essential for regulatory compliance and audits. If discrepancies in IP use are identified, they could lead to regulatory action or jeopardize the validity of the trial data.

Storage conditions are another critical aspect of investigational product management. Many investigational drugs, biologics, and devices require specific storage conditions to maintain stability, potency, and safety. Investigators are responsible for ensuring that the IP is stored under the appropriate conditions, such as temperature, humidity, and light exposure, as specified in the protocol or product label. Investigational products often require refrigeration or protection from light, and failure to store them correctly can lead to product degradation or loss of efficacy. Investigators must implement measures to monitor storage conditions, such as temperature logs or automated monitoring systems, to ensure that the IP remains within the required parameters. In the event of a storage deviation, such as a temperature excursion, the investigator must take appropriate action, which may involve consulting the sponsor to determine whether the affected IP can still be used or must be discarded.

Administration of the investigational product is a crucial responsibility for investigators and their clinical teams. Investigators must ensure that the IP is administered to participants according to the protocol's specifications, which may include specific dosing regimens, routes of administration, and timing. For example, a drug trial may require that the investigational drug be administered orally, intravenously, or through another specified route, and any deviations from this can affect both the safety of the participant and the validity of the trial data. Investigators must ensure that the clinical staff administering the IP are trained and competent in the proper procedures and follow the protocol closely.

Accurate documentation of IP administration is equally important. Investigators must maintain detailed records of each participant's exposure to the IP, including the dose, administration time, and any deviations from the protocol. This documentation is essential for ensuring protocol compliance, tracking the participant's response to the IP, and identifying any adverse reactions that may occur. In the event of a safety issue, these records provide critical information that can help investigators and sponsors determine whether the IP was administered correctly and whether the issue may be related to the IP or another factor.

The return or disposal of investigational products must be managed carefully. At the end of the trial or when a participant completes their participation, any unused IP must be returned to the sponsor or disposed of according to the sponsor's instructions. Investigators are responsible for ensuring that the IP is returned or disposed of in a manner that complies with regulatory requirements and the sponsor's specifications. This may involve documenting the return or disposal process, including the amount of IP returned or discarded and the disposal method. Proper management of IP returns and disposal is essential for maintaining regulatory compliance and ensuring the IP is not misused after the trial.

2.4 Data Integrity and Reporting

Data integrity and accurate reporting are cornerstones of ethical, scientifically sound clinical research. In the context of ICH GCP, ensuring data integrity involves meticulous attention to data collection, documentation, and reporting practices to maintain clinical trial data's accuracy, completeness, and reliability. This responsibility falls heavily on the investigator, tasked with upholding data quality in line with strict regulatory standards.

Accurate data collection starts with well-defined protocols and Case Report Forms (CRFs) that outline precise methods for capturing study data. Investigators must follow these protocols rigorously to prevent inconsistencies and errors. All data collected must reflect observations without alteration, ensuring that it genuinely represents the trial findings. In cases where corrections or clarifications are necessary, they must be appropriately documented with a clear audit trail, maintaining transparency and allowing data to be traced back to its original source.

The documentation process is another critical component of data integrity. Investigators must keep detailed records of all study-related activities and findings in source documents, the primary evidence for the trial's outcomes. Accurate documentation supports data credibility and provides a foundation for monitoring, auditing, and inspection processes.

Accurate and timely information reporting is essential for regulatory compliance and informed decision-making by sponsors, IRBs, and regulatory authorities. Investigators must ensure that reports on adverse events, protocol deviations, and periodic updates are submitted promptly and accurately represent the data.

The investigator's role in data integrity and reporting is vital for maintaining public trust in clinical research and upholding regulatory standards. By ensuring data reliability and authenticity, investigators contribute to scientifically valid outcomes and develop safe, effective patient treatments.

2.5 Communication and Collaboration

Effective communication and collaboration are essential to smooth clinical trial conduct and compliance with ICH GCP standards. Investigators, sponsors, ethics committees, and regulatory authorities must maintain open and transparent communication channels to ensure the trial's progress, address concerns, and resolve issues promptly.

Investigators are responsible for maintaining regular communication with sponsors to provide updates on study progress, report adverse events, and notify them of protocol deviations. This transparency allows the sponsor to monitor the trial's conduct and make informed decisions, ensuring the study's alignment with scientific objectives and ethical guidelines. Prompt communication with sponsors supports faster problem-solving when challenges arise, which is crucial for maintaining the trial timeline and minimizing participant risks.

The **Ethics Committee (IRB/IEC)** is a critical stakeholder safeguarding participant welfare. Investigators must inform the committee of any protocol amendments, adverse events, or significant developments that could impact participant safety or the study's ethical conduct. This ongoing interaction ensures the committee's continued oversight, supporting the ethical integrity of the trial.

Regulatory bodies like the FDA or EMA play a vital role in ensuring that clinical trials meet national and international standards. Investigators and sponsors must collaborate to meet reporting requirements, providing accurate information on trial status, safety data, and protocol changes. This collaboration enables regulatory authorities to monitor compliance, protect public health, and reinforce the credibility of clinical research.

Collaboration among these stakeholders promotes the resolution of issues promptly and enhances the overall quality of the clinical trial process. By fostering an environment of trust and cooperation, effective communication helps uphold the ethical standards of clinical research, ensuring that all parties work toward the shared goal of generating safe, effective medical knowledge.

Investigational product management is a critical component of clinical trial oversight. Investigators must ensure that the IP is handled, stored, administered, and documented appropriately to protect participants' safety and ensure the trial's scientific integrity. By maintaining rigorous accountability and documentation practices, investigators help ensure that the trial complies with GCP and regulatory requirements.

This chapter highlights the importance of an investigator's responsibilities in ensuring a clinical trial's ethical and scientifically sound conduct. From their qualifications and oversight to protecting subjects and managing investigational products, investigators play a central role in safeguarding participant safety and data integrity.

Chapter Three

Sponsor Responsibilities

3.1 Oversight and Documentation

In clinical trials, the sponsor plays a central and pivotal role, taking on ultimate responsibility for the study's design, initiation, management, and oversight. Effective oversight ensures the trial is conducted according to the approved protocol, relevant regulatory requirements, and Good Clinical Practice (GCP) guidelines. Sponsors must also ensure the integrity of the trial data and the protection of human participants. Central to the sponsor's responsibilities is maintaining accurate and comprehensive documentation, which provides an auditable trail of the trial's progress and as evidence of compliance with ethical and regulatory standards.

The oversight function of the sponsor begins well before a clinical trial is initiated. The sponsor must ensure that a scientifically sound protocol is developed, which outlines the trial's objectives, methodology, and safety measures. The protocol is the blueprint of the trial, and its development often involves collaboration between sponsors, investigators, and other stakeholders, such as statisticians, data managers, and regulatory experts. Once the protocol is finalized, it must be submitted to regulatory authorities and ethics committees for approval. The sponsor must ensure that these approvals are obtained before the trial begins, as failure to do so could lead to noncompliance with regulatory requirements.

As the trial progresses, ongoing oversight remains critical to the study's successful execution. The sponsor must ensure that the trial is conducted per the approved protocol and that any deviations are promptly identified and addressed. This is often achieved through regular communication with investigators and clinical research associates (CRAs) who monitor the trial at the site level. Monitoring activities may include reviewing data entry, source document verification, and ensuring that informed consent is obtained from all participants. Monitoring may also involve on-site visits, remote monitoring using electronic data capture (EDC) systems, and centralized monitoring approaches that analyze trial data for patterns of potential noncompliance or errors.

Sponsors are responsible for ensuring that the individuals and teams involved in monitoring the trial are adequately trained and equipped to identify and report issues that may arise during the study. This training includes protocol-specific requirements and a deep understanding of GCP principles and regulatory expectations. Sponsors must maintain comprehensive records of all monitoring activities, which provide a clear and documented trail of oversight and serve as evidence that the sponsor is fulfilling its responsibilities.

A key aspect of sponsor oversight is ensuring the proper handling and retention of essential documentation. Clinical trials generate vast amounts of data and records; the sponsor must ensure these are appropriately managed. Essential documents, such as the trial protocol, informed consent forms, monitoring reports, and regulatory approvals, must be kept in the investigator site file (ISF) and the sponsor's trial master file (TMF). These records are critical during regulatory inspections and audits, providing a transparent and auditable record of the trial's conduct.

Furthermore, the sponsor must ensure all amendments and updates to the protocol or other vital documents are handled appropriately. If changes are required, the sponsor must submit these amendments to the appropriate regulatory authorities and ethics committees for approval. Sponsors must also communicate any amendments to all trial sites and ensure that investigators implement the changes promptly. All amendments and approvals must be documented in the trial records, ensuring that the sponsor can demonstrate compliance with regulatory requirements.

The sponsor's role in oversight and documentation is multifaceted and essential for ensuring clinical trials' ethical and compliant conduct. Through effective oversight, monitoring, and meticulous documentation, the sponsor ensures the trial is conducted according to the highest scientific and ethical integrity standards.

3.2 Quality Management System

One of the most significant responsibilities of a sponsor is ensuring that a robust and effective **Quality Management System (QMS)** is in place for each clinical trial. A QMS provides a structured framework for managing and maintaining the quality of the trial, ensuring that risks to participants and data integrity are minimized. The introduction of risk-based approaches in recent years, particularly in the International Council for Harmonisation's Good Clinical Practice (ICH GCP) E6(R2) and E6(R3) revisions, has further emphasized the importance of proactive risk management and quality oversight throughout the trial lifecycle.

A QMS must encompass all aspects of trial conduct, including protocol development, monitoring, data management, and regulatory compliance. The system ensures trial processes are controlled, deviations are minimized, and issues are promptly identified and addressed. At its core, the QMS is about embedding quality into every step of the trial process rather than relying solely on inspections and audits to catch problems after they occur.

One of the critical components of a sponsor's QMS is the adoption of risk-based approaches to trial management. Traditionally, clinical trials involved extensive on-site monitoring and data verification, with equal attention paid to all trial aspects. However, this approach is resource-intensive and often inefficient, especially for large, multicenter trials. Risk-based monitoring (RBM) introduces a more strategic and focused approach, allowing sponsors to prioritize resources based on identified risks that could affect participant safety or data integrity.

RBM begins with a thorough risk assessment during the trial design phase, where potential risks are identified and evaluated based on their likelihood and impact. Common risks may include protocol deviations, data inaccuracies, or issues related to participant safety. The sponsor must then develop a risk management plan that outlines how these risks will be mitigated, monitored, and controlled throughout the trial. This plan must be continually updated as new risks emerge during the trial.

Once risks are identified, sponsors can implement targeted monitoring strategies. This might involve focusing more resources on high-risk sites or specific trial procedures while reducing oversight for lower-risk areas. For example, a sponsor may increase the frequency of monitoring visits for sites with high enrollment rates or where serious adverse events (SAEs) have been reported. Conversely, the sponsor may opt for remote monitoring or centralized data review for low-risk sites to reduce the need for on-site visits.

The sponsor's QMS should also include continuous quality improvement processes. This involves regularly reviewing the trial's performance, analyzing monitoring data, and assessing the effectiveness of risk management strategies. If issues are identified, the sponsor must be prepared to implement corrective and preventive actions (CAPA) to address the root causes and prevent similar issues from recurring. This iterative monitoring, analysis, and improvement process ensures that the trial remains on track and that any deviations or risks are promptly addressed.

Another essential element of a sponsor's QMS is training and compliance management. All trial participants, investigators, site staff, monitors, and data managers must be trained in GCP principles, protocol requirements, and specific trial procedures. The sponsor must ensure this training is documented and regularly updated as new information or amendments become available. Compliance with the training program is critical to ensure all team members understand their responsibilities and perform their duties effectively.

The sponsor must validate any technology or systems used during the trial, such as electronic data capture (EDC) systems, and meet regulatory standards for data security and integrity. This is particularly important given the increasing reliance on digital tools and decentralized trial designs, where data may be collected remotely from participants. Sponsors must have processes to ensure data is accurately captured, stored securely, and accessible only to authorized personnel.

The implementation of a Quality Management System is a fundamental responsibility of sponsors. By adopting risk-based approaches, promoting continuous quality improvement, and ensuring robust training and compliance systems, sponsors can maintain high standards of quality throughout the trial and mitigate risks to participants and data integrity. A well-implemented QMS is essential for ensuring that the trial is conducted ethically and that the results are scientifically valid.

3.3 Safety Reporting

Ensuring participant safety is the most critical responsibility of the sponsor in any clinical trial. One of the primary mechanisms through which this is achieved is safety reporting. This process involves identifying, documenting, and communicating adverse events (AEs) and other safety-related information to regulatory authorities, ethics committees, and investigators. Effective safety reporting is essential for protecting participants from harm and ensuring that regulatory authorities have the necessary information to evaluate the ongoing risk-benefit profile of the investigational product.

Adverse events are expected in clinical trials, particularly in early-phase studies where the safety profile of the investigational product is not fully understood. The sponsor is responsible for developing and implementing a system for adverse event collection and reporting that complies with GCP guidelines and regulatory requirements. This system must ensure that all AEs, regardless of their severity or relatedness to the investigational product, are captured and recorded accurately.

Serious adverse events (SAEs), which include any event that results in death, is life-threatening, requires hospitalization, or causes significant disability, must be given special attention. Sponsors are required to report SAEs to regulatory authorities and ethics committees within specific timeframes, often within 24 to 48 hours of the sponsor becoming aware of the event. The rapid reporting of SAEs ensures that regulators and ethics committees can assess whether the trial should continue or whether additional safety measures are necessary to protect participants.

Sponsors must also report **Suspected Unexpected Serious Adverse Reactions (SUSARs)**. SUSARs are adverse events that are both serious and unexpected, meaning they are not consistent with the known safety profile of the investigational product. The reporting of SUSARs is particularly critical because they may indicate a previously unknown risk associated with the investigational product. When a SUSAR is identified, the sponsor must report it to regulators and ethics committees and notify all investigators involved in the trial. This ensures that investigators can take appropriate actions, such as adjusting participant monitoring or modifying the informed consent process, to protect current and future participants from potential harm.

In some cases, safety concerns may arise that warrant immediate action by the sponsor. For example, if an unexpected safety issue is identified that poses a significant risk to participants, the sponsor may need to halt enrollment, modify the protocol, or even terminate the trial. Sponsors must be prepared to take swift action to address safety concerns and must communicate any changes to investigators, regulatory authorities, and ethics committees promptly.

An essential part of safety reporting is ongoing safety monitoring throughout the trial. Sponsors are responsible for conducting regular safety reviews, which involve analyzing AE data from all trial sites to identify patterns or trends that may indicate emerging safety concerns. This monitoring may be carried out by a data and safety monitoring board (DSMB), an independent group of experts who review safety data at predefined intervals. The DSMB has the authority to recommend trial changes, including protocol modifications or termination of the study if safety concerns arise.

Regulatory Authorities (RA) may also conduct safety reviews based on the information provided by the sponsor. Sponsors must cooperate fully with regulators during these reviews, providing them with complete and accurate safety data. If regulators identify safety concerns, they may request additional information or require the sponsor to implement new safety measures to protect participants.

To ensure that safety information is communicated effectively, sponsors must establish clear communication channels with all stakeholders involved in the trial. This includes regulatory authorities, ethics committees, investigators, and participants. Investigators must be kept informed of any new safety information, particularly if it affects the risk-benefit profile of the investigational product. Participants, too, must be informed of any new risks or safety concerns that may affect their decision to continue participating in the trial.

Safety reporting is one of the most critical aspects of a sponsor's responsibilities. By ensuring the timely and accurate reporting of adverse events, conducting ongoing safety monitoring, and swiftly addressing safety concerns, sponsors play a crucial role in protecting participants and ensuring the ethical conduct of clinical trials. Safety reporting is not only a regulatory requirement but also a fundamental ethical obligation to the participants who place their trust in the clinical research process.

3.4 Trial Design and Protocol Development

The sponsor plays a central role in developing and approving the clinical trial protocol, which is the foundation of the study's conduct, integrity, and outcomes. This responsibility includes designing a protocol that aligns with regulatory standards and meets the scientific objectives necessary to evaluate the investigational product's safety and efficacy.

Protocol development begins with the sponsor's assessment of the investigational product and its intended outcomes. The sponsor collaborates with clinical, statistical, and regulatory experts to outline the study's objectives, target population, endpoints, and methodology. Each element is carefully crafted to answer critical scientific questions, such as the product's therapeutic impact, potential side effects, and optimal dosing. This planning phase ensures the protocol's scientific validity and the feasibility of achieving meaningful results.

The sponsor must also ensure the protocol adheres to regulatory requirements from agencies such as the FDA, EMA, or other relevant authorities. This involves defining eligibility criteria, prioritizing participant safety, setting endpoints that align with clinical standards, and establishing procedures for monitoring, adverse event reporting, and data management. Adherence to these regulatory standards supports ethical study conduct and positions the investigational product for potential approval and market entry.

Once developed, the protocol undergoes rigorous internal reviews within the sponsor organization to address ethical, scientific, or operational concerns. It is then submitted to regulatory bodies and ethics committees for external review and approval. This collaborative effort, guided by ICH GCP principles, ensures that the protocol safeguards participant welfare and supports reliable, scientifically valid outcomes.

Ultimately, the sponsor's role in protocol development is crucial to balancing the trial's scientific goals with its ethical responsibility to protect participants. This results in high-quality data that contributes to public health advancements.

3.5 Investigator Selection and Support

Sponsors must select and support qualified investigators to ensure the successful conduct and integrity of a clinical trial. Investigators play a direct role in trial execution, including recruiting participants, collecting data, and ensuring participant safety. Sponsors must carefully select investigators with the requisite expertise, credentials, experience, and a commitment to Good Clinical Practice (GCP) standards.

The selection process begins with evaluating the investigator's professional qualifications, such as relevant medical or scientific expertise, experience with clinical trials, and familiarity with the therapeutic area under study. This vetting process may also involve assessing the investigator's infrastructure, including access to the necessary facilities, equipment, and staff to conduct the trial according to protocol requirements. By selecting experienced and well-equipped investigators, sponsors help ensure the quality and reliability of study data and compliance with regulatory standards.

Once selected, investigators must receive comprehensive training on the trial protocol, GCP requirements, and any specific procedures or technologies associated with the study. Sponsors are responsible for providing this training to ensure investigators understand the study's objectives, methodology, and safety procedures. Effective training helps investigators and their teams execute the study accurately and ethically, maintaining consistency across trial sites.

Throughout the trial, sponsors must offer ongoing support to investigators. This includes providing timely updates on protocol amendments, addressing queries, and supplying additional resources. Sponsors may also conduct periodic site monitoring visits to assess protocol compliance and identify improvement areas. This proactive support helps maintain data integrity, resolve issues promptly, and uphold GCP standards.

Thoroughly researching, selecting, training, and then supporting investigators will help sponsors foster an environment of trust, collaboration, and excellence, essential to achieving reliable results and safeguarding participant welfare.

This chapter has explored the critical responsibilities of sponsors in clinical trials, from oversight and documentation to quality management and safety reporting. Sponsors are essential in ensuring that trials are conducted ethically, with participant safety and data integrity at the forefront of every decision. Through meticulous oversight, robust quality management systems, and rigorous safety reporting, sponsors fulfill their role in advancing medical knowledge while protecting the rights and well-being of trial participants.

Chapter Four

Ethics and IRB/IEC Responsibilities

4.1 Independent review

Institutional Review Boards (IRBs) or Independent Ethics Committees (IECs) are indispensable in protecting human subjects participating in clinical trials. Their primary responsibility is to ensure that trials are conducted ethically, with participants' safety, rights, and welfare as the central focus. This independent review process is critical to maintaining public trust in clinical research, ensuring that studies are scientifically sound and ethically justified. IRBs and IECs are often the final checkpoint before a clinical trial can proceed, assessing protocols, informed consent documents, and potential risks or benefits to participants.

The need for independent review stems from historical abuses in clinical research, where the absence of oversight led to unethical practices that caused harm to participants. The Declaration of Helsinki, the Nuremberg Code, and other ethical frameworks emphasize the importance of independent oversight, resulting in the establishment of IRBs and IECs to review research protocols before trials begin. The independent nature of these committees ensures that they can provide unbiased and impartial evaluations, free from conflicts of interest that may arise from sponsors or investigators who have a vested interest in the trial's success.

IRBs and IECs review clinical trial protocols to ensure they are scientifically sound and ethically appropriate. The committee evaluates the potential risks and benefits, ensuring that any risks to participants are minimized and justified by the anticipated benefits. In addition to assessing scientific validity, the IRB or IEC must ensure that the study does not expose participants to unnecessary harm and that measures are in place to manage any potential risks. This balance between risk and benefit is crucial to ensuring the ethical conduct of clinical research.

In their evaluation, IRBs and IECs examine the informed consent process to ensure that participants are fully informed of the trial's purpose, procedures, potential risks, and benefits. They scrutinize the consent forms to ensure that they are written clearly and comprehensibly, avoiding technical jargon that might confuse potential participants. Furthermore, the committee ensures that participants know their right to withdraw from the trial without penalty or loss of benefits. The transparency of the informed consent process is vital to protecting the autonomy and dignity of participants, making this a critical aspect of IRB and IEC Review.

Another significant aspect of IRB and IEC oversight is ensuring that vulnerable populations, such as children, older adults, or individuals with diminished capacity to consent, are provided with additional protections. Special care must be taken to ensure that these individuals are not unduly coerced or influenced into participating in the trial and that their involvement is ethically justifiable. For example, when a trial involves pediatric participants, the IRB or IEC must ensure that parental consent is obtained and that permission is sought from the child if they can provide it. Similarly, if the trial involves participants with cognitive impairments, the committee must ensure that surrogate consent is obtained from a legally authorized representative.

Throughout the trial, the IRB or IEC maintains ongoing oversight to ensure that the trial continues to be conducted ethically. This involves regular reviews of trial progress, including any amendments to the protocol, reports of adverse events, and interim results that may affect the risk-benefit balance. The committee may require the sponsor or investigator to change the study, such as modifying the informed consent process or implementing additional safety measures, to ensure that participants remain protected.

In cases where serious ethical concerns arise, the IRB or IEC has the authority to halt or suspend the trial. This may occur if the trial is found to pose unanticipated risks to participants if the protocol is not being followed or if there are concerns about the accuracy or integrity of the data being collected. The committee's authority to stop a trial underscores its critical role in safeguarding participant welfare and ensuring that trials are conducted according to ethical principles.

IRBs and IECs are the ethical guardians of clinical research, providing an essential layer of oversight to protect human subjects. Their independent review ensures that clinical trials are conducted with the highest ethical and scientific integrity standards, helping to preserve public trust in the research process. Without their involvement, the risks to participants could go unchecked, potentially leading to unethical practices and harm to vulnerable populations.

4.2 Informed Consent Process

The informed consent process is one of the most important ethical requirements in clinical research. It ensures that participants are fully aware of the nature of the trial and voluntarily agree to participate. Informed consent is not simply a one-time event but an ongoing process that spans the entire duration of the trial, requiring transparency, clarity, and mutual understanding between the investigator and the participant. This process is central to respecting the autonomy of participants, allowing them to make informed decisions about whether or not to engage in the research.

At its core, the informed consent process protects participants' rights and dignity. It ensures that individuals are provided with all relevant information needed to make an informed decision about their participation in a clinical trial. This information includes the purpose of the study, the procedures that will be followed, the potential risks and benefits, alternative treatments (if applicable), and the participant's right to withdraw at any point without penalty. The process ensures that participants enter the study voluntarily, without coercion or undue influence, and clearly understand what their participation entails.

A critical element of informed consent is ensuring that the information provided to participants is comprehensible. The consent form must be written in a language the participant understands, avoiding technical terms or jargon that might confuse or mislead. The form must be presented at an appropriate reading level, considering the educational background and health literacy of the participant population. In some cases, sponsors may need to translate the informed consent document into different languages or provide it in alternative formats, such as audio or video, to ensure accessibility for participants with disabilities or limited literacy skills.

The presentation of information is just as important as the content of the consent document. Investigators must take the time to discuss the study with potential participants, answering any questions they may have and allowing them to reflect on the information before making a decision. It is important that participants do not feel pressured to make an immediate decision and that they are given sufficient time to consider the risks and benefits of participation. This part of the process helps ensure that consent is voluntary rather than the result of undue influence or coercion.

Informed consent is not a static process but requires continuous communication throughout the clinical trial. As the trial progresses, new information may emerge that could affect a participant's willingness to continue. For example, new risks may be identified, or the investigational product's safety profile may change. Participants must be informed of these changes when they occur, and their consent must be re-affirmed. This ongoing dialogue ensures that participants remain fully informed and can make decisions about their continued participation based on the most current information available.

Additionally, Investigators must ensure that participants understand their rights as research subjects. Participants can withdraw from the study at any time, for any reason, without facing any penalties or repercussions. They also have the right to ask questions, receive adequate medical care, and be informed of any findings that may impact their health or well-being. It is the investigator's responsibility to ensure that participants are aware of these rights and that their autonomy is respected throughout the trial.

When obtaining informed consent, investigators must also be mindful of **vulnerable populations**. Certain groups, such as children, the elderly, individuals with cognitive impairments, or economically disadvantaged individuals, may require additional protections to ensure that their consent is truly informed and voluntary. In these cases, investigators may need to obtain surrogate consent from a legally authorized representative in addition to seeking the assent of the participant. Special care must be taken to ensure that these individuals are not coerced into participating in the trial and that their participation is ethically justifiable.

The documentation of informed consent is another critical aspect of the process. Investigators must ensure that the informed consent form is properly signed and dated by both the participant and the person obtaining consent, with a copy of the form provided to the participant for their records. This documentation serves as evidence that the participant voluntarily agreed to participate in the trial after receiving and understanding all relevant information. It also provides an auditable record that can be reviewed by regulatory authorities, ethics committees, or monitors during site visits or inspections.

The informed consent process is a cornerstone of ethical clinical research. It ensures that participants have the information they need to make informed, voluntary decisions about their involvement in a study. By providing clear, comprehensive information and maintaining ongoing communication with participants, investigators help protect participants' autonomy and dignity throughout the trial. Properly conducted informed consent ensures that the research process remains transparent and accountable to both participants and regulatory bodies.

4.3 Subject Confidentiality

Protecting the confidentiality of participants is a fundamental ethical and legal obligation in clinical research. Throughout the trial, investigators and sponsors collect vast amounts of personal and medical data from participants, which must be safeguarded to ensure that individuals' privacy is maintained. Ensuring the confidentiality of participant data is not only a matter of trust but also a regulatory requirement, with guidelines such as Good Clinical Practice (GCP) and data protection laws like the General Data Protection Regulation (GDPR) in the European Union and the Health Insurance Portability and Accountability Act (HIPAA) in the United States imposing strict rules on the handling of sensitive information.

Subject confidentiality begins with the collection of personal data. When participants enroll in a clinical trial, they often provide detailed personal information, such as their medical history, demographic data, and other identifying information. This data is essential for the proper conduct of the trial, as it allows investigators to assess their eligibility, monitor their health, and evaluate the effects of the investigational product. However, the collection of this data also poses risks to participants' privacy if not handled properly.

To mitigate these risks, investigators must implement measures to ensure that personal data is anonymized or pseudonymized wherever possible. Anonymization involves removing any identifying information from the data, making it impossible to trace the information back to an individual participant. Pseudonymization, on the other hand, involves replacing identifying information with a code or identifier that can only be traced back to the participant by authorized personnel. These techniques help protect participants' privacy while allowing investigators to analyze the data for research purposes.

Access to participant data must also be carefully controlled. Only individuals who are directly involved in the trial, such as investigators, study coordinators, or monitors, should have access to personal data, and even then, access should be limited to the information that is necessary for their role in the trial. For example, a data manager responsible for analyzing trial results may not need access to participants' identities or contact details. By restricting access to personal data, investigators can reduce the risk of unauthorized disclosure or misuse of sensitive information.

Investigators must further ensure that data is stored securely throughout the trial. This may involve the use of password-protected databases, encrypted files, or secure physical storage for paper records. In the case of electronic data, investigators must ensure that the systems used to store and manage the data comply with relevant data protection regulations and security standards. This includes implementing firewalls, regular system updates, and audits to identify and address any potential vulnerabilities in the system.

Participant confidentiality also extends to the reporting of trial results. When trial data is published or shared with regulatory authorities, it must be done in a way that protects participants' identities. This often involves presenting the data in aggregate form, where individual participants cannot be identified, or using coded identifiers rather than personal information. Even in the case of adverse event reporting, where detailed information about a participant's health may need to be provided, sponsors and investigators must take care to ensure that identifying information is not disclosed.

Participants must also be informed about how their data will be used, stored, and protected. This information should be included in the informed consent process, allowing participants to make an informed decision about whether they are comfortable sharing their data for research purposes. Participants should also be informed of their rights under applicable data protection laws, such as the right to access their data, request corrections, or withdraw

4.4 Ongoing Ethical Review

The role of Institutional Review Boards (IRBs) and Independent Ethics Committees (IECs) extends beyond initial trial approval; they are continuously responsible for the ethical oversight of clinical trials. This ongoing review is essential to ensuring that trials uphold ethical standards and that participant welfare remains a top priority throughout the study.

After granting initial approval, the IRB/IEC monitors the trial by regularly reviewing safety updates, protocol amendments, and any new information that could affect participant safety or consent. These periodic assessments allow the IRB/IEC to evaluate whether the study continues to meet ethical guidelines and aligns with the principles of Good Clinical Practice (GCP). For example, IRBs/IECs may conduct scheduled reviews based on the trial's risk level or in response to specific incidents, such as adverse events or protocol deviations reported by investigators or sponsors.

The assessment of **Adverse Events (AEs)** and **Serious Adverse Events (SAEs)** is a critical aspect of the IRB/IEC'IEC'se. Investigators are required to report AEs and SAEs to the IRB/IEC, enabling the committee to assess the risk-benefit balance and determine if additional safeguards or protocol adjustments are necessary to protect participants. This vigilance is essential for promptly addressing any potential risks and adapting the study to ensure participant safety.

The IRB/IEC also reviews any protocol amendments that may impact the study's design aspects, such as changes in the participant population, dosing, or study procedures. By reviewing these amendments, the IRB/IEC ensures that participants are adequately informed of any modifications and that their consent remains valid under the revised conditions.

The IRB/IEC's ethical review is fundamental to the trial's integrity. By continuously monitoring the study, the IRB/IEC provides an added layer of protection for participants and reinforces public trust in the ethical conduct of clinical research.

4.5 Risk-Benefit Assessment

A key responsibility of the Institutional Review Board (IRB) and Independent Ethics Committee (IEC) is to conduct a comprehensive risk-benefit assessment for clinical trials. This process evaluates the potential risks to participants against the anticipated benefits, ensuring that the trial is ethically justified and that participant welfare is prioritized. The IRB/IEC's ongoing review of this balance is essential to maintaining ethical standards throughout the study's duration.

During the initial review, the IRB/IEC assesses the trial's objectives, design, and methodology to identify any foreseeable risks to participants. This includes evaluating the investigational product profile, the invasiveness of study procedures, and any physical or psychological burdens on participants. The committee considers these risks relative to the potential benefits, including advancing medical knowledge, providing participants access to potentially beneficial treatments, or contributing to public health improvements.

The IRB/IEC also involves ensuring that the trial design minimizes risks wherever possible. This may include recommending alternative procedures that are less invasive, reducing study-related burdens, or requiring additional safeguards for vulnerable populations. The IRB/IEC may suggest modifications to the protocol that align with ethical standards while preserving the trial's scientific validity.

The assessment does not end at initial approval; the IRB/IEC conducts periodic reviews to reevaluate the risk-benefit ratio in light of new data. If adverse events or other concerns arise, the committee reassesses whether the benefits still justify the risks. This dynamic approach allows the IRB/IEC to respond proactively, requesting protocol adjustments or even halting the trial if risks become unacceptably high.

The IRB/IEC diligently balances risks and benefits and helps ensure that clinical trials contribute positively to scientific knowledge and participant health. It safeguards participants and upholds the ethical integrity of the research process.

This chapter emphasizes the ethical framework in clinical trials, highlighting the critical roles of independent reviews by IRBs/IECs, informed consent, subject confidentiality, ongoing oversight, and risk-benefit assessment. These processes collectively ensure participant safety, ethical compliance, and the integrity of clinical research.

Chapter Five

Computerized and Digital Systems

5.1 Implementation and Use of Computerized Systems in Clinical Trials

As clinical trials embrace advanced technologies, integrating computerized and digital systems is becoming fundamental to trial operations. These systems are indispensable in managing vast amounts of trial data, enhancing efficiency, improving accuracy, and ensuring compliance with the latest regulatory standards. The ICH GCP E6(R3) guidelines underscore the critical role of computerized systems, emphasizing that they must be designed and used to guarantee data integrity, participant safety, and regulatory compliance. This chapter will delve into the proper implementation, validation, and management of these systems, focusing on the security measures required to protect trial data and participants.

The ICH GCP E6(R3) guidelines emphasize that implementing computerized systems in clinical trials must follow a structured, compliant approach that aligns with the study's objectives, operational needs, and regulatory requirements. These systems, which range from electronic data capture (EDC) platforms to interactive response technology (IRT) for managing randomization and drug supply, play a critical role in every clinical trial stage—from participant enrollment to data collection, monitoring, and analysis.

A rigorous assessment is required before implementation to ensure that these systems are fit for purpose. This assessment includes confirming that the system is compatible with existing infrastructure, has adequate functionality to meet trial needs, and can be securely integrated with other tools used in the study, such as **Laboratory Information Management Systems (LIMS)** or **Electronic Medical Records (EMRs).** The selected system should align with Good Clinical Practice (GCP) principles, focusing on accuracy, reliability, and trial data protection.

User access control is one of the most critical considerations in implementing computerized systems. The ICH GCP E6(R3) guidelines require that all computerized systems used in clinical trials have robust security protocols that restrict access to authorized personnel only. This means that each user must have a unique login credential, and their access to specific system parts should be aligned with their role in the trial. For instance, clinical investigators may need full access to participant records and data entry fields, while data managers may only require access to data review and statistical analysis functions. **Role-Based Access Control (RBAC)** ensures that individuals can only access the data and functionality necessary for their responsibilities, significantly reducing the risk of data breaches or unauthorized modifications.

Another critical aspect of implementing computerized systems is the development of **Standard Operating Procedures (SOPs)**. SOPs ensure that all users understand how to interact with the system, how data should be entered and managed, and how to troubleshoot common issues. SOPs should be clearly documented and regularly updated to reflect changes in the system or trial processes. Moreover, all personnel interacting with the system must be adequately trained. This training should include not only the operational aspects of the system but also a clear understanding of regulatory requirements, including GCP guidelines and data protection laws such as **GDPR** or **HIPAA**. Regular training assessments help confirm that users continue to adhere to these standards throughout the trial.

The successful implementation of computerized systems in clinical trials hinges on selecting systems that meet trial-specific needs, enforcing stringent user access controls, developing comprehensive SOPs, and ensuring adequate personnel training. These measures are essential to maintaining trial data's accuracy, security, and reliability.

5.2 Validation and Compliance of Digital Systems

Validation of computerized systems is critical to ensure they function as intended and meet all regulatory expectations. According to ICH GCP E6(R3), system validation is required before the system can be deployed in a clinical trial. Validation processes must confirm that the system produces accurate, reliable data consistently and adheres to all relevant regulatory standards. System validation is not a one-time task but an ongoing process, especially as systems are updated or modified during a trial.

The validation process begins with functional testing to ensure all system parts work according to the predefined requirements. This includes testing features such as data entry fields, audit trails, and export functions. The system must also be validated under real-world trial conditions to confirm that it can handle the expected volume of data and user interactions without performance degradation.

ICH GCP E6(R3) emphasizes that validation should include the system's ability to maintain data integrity through automatic data validation checks, which can flag missing or inconsistent data, and real-time alerts for data discrepancies. Systems must also have audit trails, critical for maintaining transparency and accountability. The audit trail records every change made to the data, including what was changed, by whom, and when. This documentation ensures that any alterations to the data are fully traceable and that the data can be reconstructed if necessary for audits or inspections.

Regulatory compliance is another crucial element of computerized systems validation. Systems used in clinical trials must comply with relevant data protection regulations, such as **GDPR (General Data Protection Regulation)** in Europe or **HIPAA (Health Insurance Portability and Accountability Act)** in the U.S. These regulations mandate that participant data is securely stored, transmitted, and accessed only by authorized individuals. System validation must confirm that appropriate encryption measures are in place to protect sensitive participant information at rest and during transmission. Encryption ensures that even if data is intercepted, it cannot be read or used without the proper decryption key.

These systems must also include user authentication protocols to ensure that only authorized personnel can access the system. This might include multi-factor authentication (MFA), which requires users to verify their identity through two or more independent factors, such as a password and a verification code sent to their phone. MFA significantly enhances system security by reducing the risk of unauthorized access.

The validation process also involves regular system audits to ensure ongoing compliance. These audits verify that the system continues to function correctly, that security protocols remain effective, and that any updates to the system do not compromise its integrity. In cases where significant changes are made to the system, revalidation may be required to confirm that the system continues to meet all regulatory and operational requirements.

System validation is a critical process that ensures computerized systems in clinical trials are compliant, reliable, and capable of maintaining data integrity. It involves rigorous testing, regulatory compliance checks, encryption, user authentication, and regular audits to maintain the system's integrity throughout the trial.

5.3 Data Integrity and Management in Digital Environments

Data integrity is central to the success of any clinical trial, and the ICH GCP E6(R3) guidelines emphasize maintaining the accuracy, completeness, and consistency of data in digital environments. Computerized systems must be designed and used to guarantee the integrity of the data collected, ensuring that trial results are scientifically valid and can withstand regulatory scrutiny.

One of the primary mechanisms for ensuring data integrity is the use of automated data validation checks within the system. These checks can identify and flag real-time errors, such as out-of-range values, missing data, or inconsistent entries. For example, if a participant's age is entered as "150," the system should automatically flag this as an error and prompt the user to correct the entry. Similarly, if critical data points—such as vital signs or laboratory results—are missing, the system should alert the user to fill in the required information before the data can be finalized.

An audit trail is another crucial feature of computerized systems for maintaining data integrity. The audit trail documents the system's actions, including data entries, modifications, and deletions. It records who made each change, what was changed, and when. This level of transparency is essential for ensuring that any alterations to the data are justified and traceable. Audit trails are significant during audits and inspections, as they provide a detailed record of how the data was handled throughout the trial.

Maintaining the integrity of data also requires the implementation of data backup and recovery plans. Clinical trials generate large volumes of critical data, and the loss or corruption of this data can have catastrophic consequences for the trial. To mitigate this risk, sponsors must develop robust backup systems that store copies of the trial data in secure, off-site locations. Backup data should be encrypted to protect it from unauthorized access, and regular testing of the recovery process is essential to ensure that data can be restored quickly and accurately in the event of a system failure, cyberattack, or other external threat.

Data security is an area of increasing focus in the ICH GCP E6(R3) guidelines, given the rising threat of cyberattacks and data breaches in the healthcare and research sectors. Clinical trials handle sensitive participant information, and any data breach can have profound ethical and legal implications. To protect data from unauthorized access, systems must employ encryption protocols both when data is at rest (stored on servers or devices) and during transmission (when data is transferred between systems or users). Encryption ensures that even if data is intercepted or stolen, it cannot be read or used without the correct decryption key.

Additionally, firewalls, intrusion detection systems, and regular vulnerability assessments should be implemented to protect the system from cyberattacks. Firewalls prevent unauthorized access to the system, while intrusion detection systems monitor network traffic for signs of suspicious activity. Regular vulnerability assessments help identify and address potential security weaknesses before malicious actors can exploit them.

When storing digital data, technical security measures and physical security must also be considered. Servers and other hardware used to store trial data should be located in secure, access-controlled environments. Only authorized personnel should have physical access to these systems, and security protocols such as biometric access or keycard systems can be used to control entry.

Finally, sponsors and investigators must ensure they comply with data protection laws, such as GDPR and HIPAA, which require stringent safeguards for handling personal health information. Participants must be informed about how their data will be used, stored, and protected, and they must consent to the collection and processing of their data. Regular audits and reviews of data security protocols are essential for ensuring ongoing compliance with these regulations.

In conclusion, maintaining data integrity and security in digital environments is paramount to clinical trials' success and ethical conduct. By implementing automated data validation checks, audit trails, backup systems, and robust security protocols, sponsors and investigators can ensure trial data is accurate, complete, and protected from unauthorized access. These measures are critical for upholding the scientific validity of the trial and safeguarding participant confidentiality.

5.4 Security and Access Control

Security and access control are critical components in managing clinical trial data, especially as digital systems and electronic data capture (EDC) become standard practice. Protecting sensitive participant information and trial data integrity requires stringent security protocols and access management strategies. These measures safeguard participant confidentiality and support regulatory compliance and data reliability.

Digital security in clinical trials relies on implementing advanced encryption methods to protect data both at rest and in transit. Encryption ensures that sensitive information remains secure and unreadable to unauthorized parties, even if data is intercepted or compromised. Additionally, secure data storage solutions, including cloud-based servers with robust security certifications, provide an extra layer of protection against potential breaches.

Access control is equally crucial in managing who can view, edit, or export trial data. Proper authorization protocols ensure that only authorized personnel—those directly involved in the study—can access sensitive information. Role-based access control (RBAC) systems are commonly used to limit access based on user roles, ensuring that each team member has only the level of access necessary for their responsibilities. This approach minimizes the risk of data manipulation or unauthorized access, supporting data integrity and compliance.

Audit trails are also essential for tracking access to trial data. Audit trails create a transparent record that can be reviewed in case of discrepancies or during audits by documenting every instance of data access, modification, or deletion. This traceability reinforces accountability within the trial team and allows for quick identification of potential issues.

Implementing robust security and access control measures aligns with Good Clinical Practice (GCP) standards and regulatory expectations. It ensures participant confidentiality and that trial data remain accurate and trustworthy. Together, these practices form a secure environment that upholds clinical research's ethical and scientific integrity.

Computerized and digital systems have become integral to modern clinical trials, enabling more efficient data collection, processing, and storage. However, using these systems requires careful implementation, rigorous validation, and robust data management processes to ensure compliance with the ICH GCP E6(R3) guidelines. By focusing on system security, data integrity, and regulatory compliance, sponsors and investigators can ensure that their clinical trials are conducted with the highest standards of quality and accountability.

This chapter discusses the critical role of computerized systems in clinical trials, highlighting their implementation, validation, and security measures to ensure data integrity, regulatory compliance, and participant confidentiality. It underscores the importance of robust audit trails, access controls, and proactive system monitoring to uphold clinical research's ethical and scientific standards.

Chapter Six

Monitoring and Auditing

6.1 Purpose of Monitoring

The purpose of monitoring in clinical trials is multifaceted, playing a crucial role in maintaining the quality, integrity, and safety of the study. Monitoring serves as a mechanism to ensure that the trial is conducted in compliance with the protocol, Good Clinical Practice (GCP) guidelines, and regulatory requirements. It is designed to protect the rights and well-being of participants while ensuring the accuracy, completeness, and credibility of the data generated during the trial. By regularly visiting trial sites and conducting reviews, monitors help identify potential issues early, enabling timely corrective actions to prevent protocol deviations, data discrepancies, or safety concerns from compromising the trial.

Monitoring activities begin as soon as the trial is initiated and continue until its conclusion. **Site initiation Visits (SIV)** mark the first step in the monitoring process, where the monitor, also known as a **Clinical Research Associate (CRA)**, visits the trial site to ensure that all preparatory steps have been completed before the study begins. During this visit, the CRA confirms that the site has the necessary approvals from ethics committees and regulatory authorities, verifies that the investigator and staff have received adequate training on the protocol and GCP guidelines, and ensures that the investigational product has been received and stored under the appropriate conditions. The site initiation visit sets the stage for the trial's smooth conduct, helping to ensure that the site is prepared to enroll participants and collect data according to the protocol.

Once the trial is underway, routine monitoring visits are conducted to assess the ongoing conduct of the study. These visits allow the monitor to review the site's progress in enrolling participants, evaluate the completeness and accuracy of data collection, and ensure that participants' safety is being adequately protected. One of the primary tasks of the monitor during these visits is to perform **Source Data Verification (SDV)**, which involves cross-checking data entered into **Case Report Forms (CRFs)** with the original source documents, such as medical records, laboratory results, or patient diaries. This process is essential for ensuring that the data entered into the study database is accurate and reliable, as discrepancies between the source data and the CRFs can compromise the integrity of the trial's findings. Monitors also review the site's regulatory documents, such as informed consent forms and ethics committee approvals, to ensure that they are up to date and in compliance with regulatory requirements.

Monitors are also responsible for assessing protocol compliance during their visits. This involves ensuring that the site is following the protocol's procedures for participant enrollment, treatment administration, and data collection. For example, the monitor may review participant records to confirm that eligibility criteria are being adhered to, that the investigational product is being administered according to the protocol's specifications, and that any deviations from the protocol are promptly documented and reported. Ensuring protocol compliance is critical for maintaining the scientific validity of the trial, as deviations can introduce bias or confound the study's results.

One of the key purposes of monitoring is to protect participant safety. Monitors assess whether the site is following appropriate procedures for obtaining informed consent, reporting adverse events, and providing medical care to participants. They review the site's records of adverse events (AEs) and serious adverse events (SAEs) to ensure that these events are being reported to the sponsor and regulatory authorities in a timely manner. Monitors also evaluate the site's processes for managing participant safety, such as whether participants are being monitored for potential side effects of the investigational product and whether appropriate medical interventions are being provided if needed.

In addition to on-site visits, monitoring may also involve remote monitoring activities, particularly in trials that utilize electronic data capture (EDC) systems. Remote monitoring allows CRAs to review data entered into the study database from a distance, identifying potential discrepancies or issues without the need for a physical visit to the site. While remote monitoring cannot replace the thoroughness of an on-site visit, it serves as a valuable tool for detecting data anomalies or protocol deviations between routine visits, enabling more timely interventions.

The purpose of monitoring in clinical trials is to ensure that the study is conducted in accordance with the protocol, GCP, and regulatory requirements while safeguarding participant safety and data integrity. Through regular site visits and ongoing reviews, monitors help identify potential issues early, allowing for corrective actions that protect the quality of the trial and the validity of its results.

6.2 Risk-Based Monitoring (RBM)

Risk-Based Monitoring (RBM) is an innovative approach to trial oversight that has revolutionized the way clinical trials are monitored. Traditional monitoring methods, which involved frequent and exhaustive on-site visits to all trial sites, were resource-intensive, time-consuming, and often inefficient, particularly for large multicenter trials. RBM offers a more targeted and efficient alternative by focusing monitoring efforts on the areas of the trial that pose the greatest risks to participant safety and data integrity. This approach allows sponsors and monitors to allocate resources more strategically, ensuring that the most critical aspects of the trial receive the attention they need while reducing unnecessary monitoring activities in lower-risk areas.

The foundation of RBM lies in a comprehensive risk assessment conducted during the trial's planning phase. The goal of this assessment is to identify potential risks that could impact participants' safety or the trial data's reliability and to develop strategies for mitigating those risks. Risks may be associated with various aspects of the trial, including the protocol's complexity, the investigative sites' experience, the study population's characteristics, or the nature of the investigational product. For example, a trial involving a high-risk population, such as elderly patients with multiple comorbidities, may require more intensive monitoring of safety data, while a trial with a complex dosing regimen may require closer scrutiny of protocol compliance.

Once risks have been identified, the sponsor and monitors can develop a risk management plan that outlines the specific monitoring activities that will be implemented to address each risk. This plan serves as a roadmap for the RBM approach, detailing how monitoring resources will be allocated and what strategies will be used to manage the identified risks. For instance, the plan may specify that high-enrolling sites will receive more frequent on-site visits, while sites with low enrollment or no significant deviations may be monitored remotely. The plan may also include centralized monitoring activities, such as statistical analyses of data trends across sites, to detect potential issues that may not be immediately apparent through traditional monitoring methods.

A key advantage of RBM is its flexibility. Unlike traditional monitoring, which typically follows a fixed schedule of site visits regardless of the trial's progress or risk profile, RBM allows monitoring activities to be adapted as the trial evolves. As new risks emerge or existing risks are mitigated, the monitoring plan can be adjusted accordingly. For example, if a site is identified as having a high rate of protocol deviations, the sponsor may increase the frequency of on-site visits to that site while reducing monitoring at other sites that are performing well. Conversely, if a site demonstrates consistent compliance with the protocol and has no significant issues, the sponsor may reduce the intensity of monitoring at that site, freeing up resources for higher-risk areas.

RBM also emphasizes the use of centralized monitoring tools, which allow sponsors and monitors to analyze data across all sites in real-time. Centralized monitoring involves the use of statistical and data analytics tools to detect patterns or trends in the data that may indicate potential issues, such as unusually high rates of adverse events at a particular site or discrepancies in the timing of data entry. By identifying these trends early, sponsors can take proactive steps to address potential problems before they escalate. For example, if a centralized monitoring analysis reveals that one site has a higher-than-expected rate of protocol deviations, the sponsor may conduct a targeted on-site visit to investigate the issue and implement corrective actions.

One of the most significant benefits of RBM is its ability to enhance data quality while reducing the burden on both sponsors and investigative sites. By focusing monitoring efforts on the areas of greatest risk, RBM helps ensure that critical data points, such as primary efficacy and safety endpoints, are closely monitored, while less critical aspects of the trial are monitored less intensively. This targeted approach not only improves the overall quality of the data but also reduces the administrative burden on site staff, who may otherwise be overwhelmed by frequent and exhaustive monitoring visits. RBM also reduces the cost of monitoring by allowing sponsors to prioritize resources based on risk rather than conducting blanket monitoring activities across all sites.

However, RBM is not without its challenges. One of the key difficulties in implementing RBM is the need for robust data management systems that can support real-time data analysis and centralized monitoring activities. Sponsors must invest in advanced technology platforms that can capture, store, and analyze data from multiple sites in real time while ensuring that the data is accurate, complete, and secure. Additionally, the success of RBM depends on the ability of sponsors and monitors to conduct thorough risk assessments and to adapt their monitoring strategies as the trial progresses. This requires ongoing communication and collaboration between sponsors, monitors, and investigative sites, as well as a commitment to continuous improvement in monitoring practices.

Risk-Based Monitoring represents a paradigm shift in clinical trial oversight, offering a more efficient, flexible, and targeted approach to ensuring trial quality and participant safety. By focusing monitoring efforts on the areas of greatest risk, RBM allows sponsors to optimize resource allocation, enhance data quality, and reduce the burden on investigative sites while maintaining the highest standards of compliance with regulatory requirements. As technology continues to advance and data analytics tools become more sophisticated, RBM is likely to play an increasingly important role in the future of clinical trial monitoring.

6.3 Auditing Practices

Auditing is a critical aspect of clinical trial oversight, providing an independent and systematic evaluation of trial conduct, data integrity, and compliance with regulatory requirements and GCP guidelines. While monitoring focuses on the day-to-day conduct of the trial, auditing serves as a more comprehensive and retrospective review, examining whether the trial has been conducted in accordance with the approved protocol, applicable regulations, and ethical standards. Audits are typically conducted by the sponsor or an external auditor, and their primary purpose is to identify non-compliance, deficiencies, or areas for improvement in the trial's conduct, with the goal of ensuring that the study meets the highest standards of quality and integrity.

One of the key functions of an audit is to verify compliance with ICH GCP guidelines, which set the international standard for the ethical and scientific conduct of clinical trials. During an audit, the auditor reviews a wide range of trial-related documents and activities, including the trial protocol, informed consent process, source data, CRFs, and regulatory approvals. The audit process involves thoroughly examining both the sponsor's and investigator's responsibilities, ensuring that all trial activities are conducted per GCP principles. For example, the auditor may review the site's informed consent forms to verify that participants were properly informed about the trial's risks and benefits and that consent was obtained before any study-related procedures were initiated.

Audits also assess the accuracy and integrity of the trial data. This involves comparing the data entered into the study database with the original source documents to ensure that the data is complete, accurate, and consistent. For example, the auditor may review participants' medical records to verify that the data on adverse events, concomitant medications, or laboratory results recorded in the CRFs accurately reflect the information in the source documents. Auditors also assess whether the data has been entered into the study database in a timely manner and whether any discrepancies or missing data have been appropriately addressed. Data integrity is critical for ensuring that the trial's findings are reliable and can be used to support regulatory approval or scientific publications.

Auditing practices also play a key role in identifying protocol deviations and violations. While monitors may detect deviations during routine site visits, audits provide a more comprehensive and retrospective review of the trial's conduct, allowing auditors to identify patterns of non-compliance that may not be immediately apparent during monitoring. For example, an audit may reveal that a site has consistently failed to adhere to the protocol's eligibility criteria, enrolling participants who do not meet the inclusion or exclusion criteria. In such cases, the auditor will document the deviations and assess their impact on the trial's overall validity. If the deviations are found to have compromised participant safety or data integrity, the sponsor may be required to implement corrective actions, such as retraining site staff or revising the protocol.

Auditing is also a key tool for identifying systemic issues that may affect the conduct of the trial across multiple sites. For example, an audit may reveal that multiple sites are experiencing difficulties with data entry, resulting in delays in submitting CRFs or inconsistencies in the data being collected. In such cases, the auditor may recommend that the sponsor implement additional training or support for site staff or that the data management process be revised to address the underlying issues. By identifying these systemic problems, audits help sponsors improve the overall quality of the trial and ensure that issues are addressed before they escalate.

Regulatory compliance is another critical focus of auditing practices. Auditors assess whether the trial has been conducted in accordance with applicable regulatory requirements, including those related to participant safety, data management, and reporting. For example, the auditor may review the site's procedures for reporting SAEs to ensure that they are being reported to the sponsor and regulatory authorities within the required timeframes. Auditors also assess whether the site has maintained all necessary regulatory documents, such as ethics committee approvals and investigator agreements, and whether these documents are up to date and properly filed. Non-compliance with regulatory requirements can result in significant penalties, including the suspension or termination of the trial, making it essential for sponsors and investigators to ensure that they are fully compliant with all applicable regulations.

Audits are not limited to on-site visits but may also involve centralized audits or remote audits, particularly in trials that use electronic data capture systems. In a centralized audit, the auditor reviews data and documents from multiple sites from a central location, using statistical and data analytics tools to identify potential issues. Remote audits, on the other hand, involve reviewing electronic records and conducting interviews with site staff via teleconferencing or other remote communication tools. These approaches allow auditors to assess the conduct of the trial without the need for physical visits to each site, making them a valuable tool for large multicenter trials or trials conducted in geographically dispersed locations.

Auditing is a critical component of clinical trial oversight, providing an independent and comprehensive evaluation of the trial's conduct, data integrity, and compliance with regulatory requirements and GCP guidelines. By identifying non-compliance, deficiencies, or areas for improvement, audits help sponsors and investigators ensure that the trial meets the highest standards of quality and integrity. Through a combination of on-site visits, centralized audits, and remote audits, auditors provide valuable insights that help safeguard participant safety, ensure data reliability, and maintain regulatory compliance.

6.4 Investigator and Site Performance Evaluation

Evaluating the performance of investigators and study sites is a vital part of clinical trial oversight. It ensures that the trial is conducted in accordance with the protocol, regulatory standards, and Good Clinical Practice (GCP) guidelines. Effective performance evaluation contributes to data quality, participant safety, and timely completion of the trial, all of which are essential for the credibility and reliability of trial outcomes.

Adherence to the protocol is a primary focus of performance evaluation. Investigators and sites are responsible for executing study procedures as outlined in the protocol, which includes participant recruitment, informed consent, and data collection. Regular site monitoring visits and centralized data reviews help assess whether these activities are performed accurately and consistently. Any deviations from the protocol, whether in procedures or data collection, are identified promptly and addressed to maintain data integrity and compliance.

Quality standards are further evaluated through monitoring visits, audits, and performance metrics. Key performance indicators (KPIs) such as enrollment rates, data entry timeliness, and accuracy provide a quantitative measure of site performance. Sites that consistently meet these standards demonstrate a commitment to quality, while those that fall short may require additional support, training, or corrective action to bring them in line with trial expectations.

Timely issue resolution is another critical component of site evaluation. Clinical trials often encounter challenges, including recruitment delays, adverse events, or protocol deviations. Evaluating how quickly and effectively a site addresses these issues reflects its overall capability to maintain compliance and participant safety. Sponsors and Clinical Research Organizations (CROs) work closely with sites to facilitate prompt resolution, ensuring that the trial progresses smoothly and adheres to regulatory requirements.

Sponsors and CROs uphold the standards necessary for producing valid, high-quality data, reinforcing the ethical and scientific foundations of clinical research by thoroughly and regularly evaluating investigator and site performance.

6.5 Corrective and Preventive Actions (CAPA)

Corrective and Preventive Actions (CAPA) play an essential role in maintaining compliance and enhancing the quality of clinical trials. CAPA involves a structured approach to identify, investigate, and resolve issues found during monitoring, audits, or inspections, with the ultimate goal of preventing recurrence and improving trial conduct. This process aligns with Good Clinical Practice (GCP) standards and is crucial for meeting regulatory expectations.

The identification of issues typically begins during routine monitoring visits, audits, or data reviews, where non-compliance, protocol deviations or quality concerns may be uncovered. Once an issue is detected, it is essential to perform a thorough root cause analysis to understand why the issue occurred. This analysis allows the study team to implement not only corrective actions but also preventive measures to address the underlying cause and prevent similar issues in the future.

Corrective actions are immediate steps taken to resolve identified issues, such as retraining site staff, updating procedures, or adjusting data management practices. These actions aim to restore compliance quickly and mitigate any potential impact on trial integrity or participant safety.

On the other hand, preventive actions focus on long-term improvements to reduce the likelihood of recurring issues. For example, if a protocol deviation occurred due to unclear instructions, a preventive action might involve revising the protocol for clarity or enhancing training materials for site personnel.

Effective CAPA implementation includes documenting each step, from issue identification and root cause analysis to corrective and preventive measures. This documentation serves as an essential record for regulatory bodies, demonstrating that the trial is conducted responsibly and that continuous improvements are made.

By integrating CAPA into trial management, sponsors and Clinical Research Organizations (CROs) can ensure ongoing compliance, reinforce data quality, and uphold ethical standards, all of which are essential to the success and integrity of clinical research.

This chapter has explored the key aspects of monitoring and auditing in clinical trials, highlighting their roles in ensuring trial quality, data integrity, and participant safety. Through regular site visits, risk-based monitoring, and comprehensive auditing practices, sponsors and investigators can maintain the highest standards of compliance and ethical conduct, ensuring the success of the trial and the protection of the participants involved.

Chapter Seven

Data Handling and Record Management

7.1 Data Integrity

In clinical trials, the integrity of the data collected is fundamental to the credibility of the study's results. Ensuring data integrity means that the data is accurate, complete, consistent, and reliable throughout the lifecycle of the trial—from collection and processing to analysis and storage. Data integrity is essential for drawing scientifically valid conclusions, complying with regulatory requirements, and ensuring that any investigational product can be evaluated properly for safety and efficacy. Without data integrity, the findings of a clinical trial can be rendered invalid, leading to compromised patient safety and unreliable conclusions about the investigational product.

To ensure data accuracy, all data entered into the system must precisely reflect the original observations made during the trial. This includes measurements, clinical assessments, patient responses, and other relevant trial data. One of the key ways to ensure accuracy is through source data verification (SDV), a process in which data entered into Case Report Forms (CRFs) is cross-checked against the original source documents, such as medical records, laboratory results, or patient-reported diaries. SDV is a critical aspect of trial monitoring and helps ensure that what is recorded in the study database represents what occurred during the trial.

The completeness of data is another critical component of data integrity. All relevant data points must be collected for every participant in accordance with the trial protocol. Missing or incomplete data can significantly undermine the reliability of the trial's results. Therefore, investigators must ensure that all required fields in the CRFs are filled out and that no critical information is omitted. This includes timely collection of laboratory results, adverse event reports, and patient outcomes. A thorough and complete dataset allows for proper statistical analysis and ensures that the study's findings are robust and reliable.

Consistency is also key to data integrity. Data should be collected consistently across all trial sites, with adherence to the protocol and standard operating procedures (SOPs). For example, if a particular laboratory test is required at specific time points during the trial, it is essential that all sites follow the same procedures and timeframes for testing. Inconsistent data collection can introduce variability that may bias the results and reduce the study's ability to detect the true effect of the investigational product. Data collection tools, such as CRFs and electronic data capture (EDC) systems, must be standardized across all sites to ensure consistency in the information recorded.

Reliability is the final element of data integrity and relates to the ability to trust the data generated in the study. Reliable data is reproducible, meaning the results would be similar if the same trial were conducted under the same conditions. Reliability is ensured through strict adherence to the trial protocol, SOPs, and GCP guidelines and rigorous training of all personnel involved in data collection and management. Quality control measures, such as audit trails, regular monitoring, and data validation, help ensure that data is reliable and that any errors or discrepancies are promptly identified and corrected.

One key aspect of ensuring data integrity in modern clinical trials is the use of electronic data capture (EDC) systems. These systems allow for real-time data entry and monitoring, reducing the potential for transcription errors and improving data accuracy. EDC systems often have built-in validation checks that can alert site staff to potential data entry errors, such as out-of-range values or missing fields, which can then be corrected before the data is finalized. Additionally, EDC systems provide an audit trail that tracks every modification made to the data, ensuring transparency and accountability in the data handling process.

Data integrity also extends to the security and confidentiality of the data. Investigators must ensure that participant data is protected from unauthorized access and that all data is handled in accordance with applicable data protection regulations, such as the General Data Protection Regulation (GDPR) in the European Union or the Health Insurance Portability and Accountability Act (HIPAA) in the United States. Data should be stored in secure, password-protected databases, and access should be limited to authorized personnel. Maintaining data confidentiality not only protects participants' privacy but also upholds the ethical standards of the trial.

Data integrity is essential for ensuring the validity and reliability of clinical trial results. By focusing on accuracy, completeness, consistency, and reliability and implementing strong data management systems, investigators can ensure that the data collected during the trial is of the highest quality. This, in turn, supports the ethical conduct of the trial and provides a solid foundation for evaluating the investigational product's safety and efficacy.

7.2 Source Data and Case Report Forms (CRFs)

The proper management of source data and Case Report Forms (CRFs) is a critical aspect of data handling in clinical trials. Source data refers to the original information recorded about participants during the trial, such as medical records, laboratory results, and patient-reported outcomes. CRFs, on the other hand, are the structured forms used to capture trial-specific data, which is later transferred into the study database for analysis. Ensuring that source data and CRFs are accurate, complete, and properly aligned is essential for maintaining the integrity of the trial data and supporting the study's conclusions.

Source data serves as the foundation of the trial's data, providing the first record of observations made during the study. This data may include various types of records, such as physician notes, hospital charts, diagnostic reports, patient diaries, and electronic health records. Source data is essential because it provides a traceable and verifiable record of the information collected during the trial, allowing monitors and auditors to cross-check the accuracy of the data entered into the CRFs. The integrity of source data is fundamental to the credibility of the trial's findings, as any discrepancies between source data and CRFs can call the validity of the study into question.

It is vital that source data is accurately and contemporaneously recorded. Investigators must ensure that all observations, clinical findings, and other relevant information are recorded at the time they occur, as retrospective data entry can lead to inaccuracies or the omission of critical details. For example, if a patient experiences an adverse event during the trial, the details of that event must be recorded immediately, including the date, time, severity, and any actions taken in response. Delayed or incomplete recording of source data can result in missing or unreliable information, which can compromise the safety of participants and the validity of the trial's results.

Once the source data is recorded, it must be transferred into the Case Report Forms (CRFs), which are the primary data collection tools used in clinical trials. CRFs are designed to capture all relevant information about the participants' experiences during the trial, including demographic data, medical history, laboratory results, and treatment outcomes. The CRFs provide a standardized format for recording data, ensuring that the information is collected consistently across all trial sites. This consistency is crucial for enabling the comparison of data between different participants and sites, which is essential for conducting statistical analyses and drawing valid conclusions.

The process of entering data into CRFs must be done with meticulous attention to detail to ensure accuracy and completeness. Each data point entered into the CRFs must exactly match the information recorded in the source documents, with no discrepancies or omissions. Any corrections or changes made to the CRFs must be clearly documented, with a justification for the change and the person's signature. In electronic CRFs (eCRFs), audit trails automatically track any modifications made to the data, providing a transparent record of all changes.

To ensure that the CRFs accurately reflect the source data, monitors perform source data verification (SDV) during site visits. SDV involves cross-checking the data entered into the CRFs with the original source documents to confirm that the information is accurate and complete. For example, if a patient's blood pressure reading is recorded in the source data as 120/80 mmHg, the monitor will verify that the same reading is entered into the CRFs without any discrepancies. SDV is an essential quality control measure that helps ensure the reliability of the trial data and identifies any errors or inconsistencies that need to be corrected.

Maintaining the confidentiality of source data and CRFs is also very important. Both source data and CRFs contain sensitive information about participants, including their medical history and personal identifiers. Investigators must implement strict confidentiality measures to protect this information from unauthorized access. Source documents should be stored in secure, locked locations, and electronic CRFs should be password-protected and encrypted. Access to these records should be limited to authorized personnel only, and all data handling procedures must comply with applicable data protection regulations, such as GDPR and HIPAA.

Another important consideration is the retention of source data and CRFs. Regulatory authorities require that all source documents and CRFs be retained for a specified period after the conclusion of the trial, to allow for regulatory inspections, audits, or reanalysis of the data if necessary. The exact duration of the retention period varies depending on local regulations, but it is typically several years. Investigators must ensure that these records are stored securely and remain accessible throughout the retention period.

The proper handling of source data and CRFs is critical to the success of a clinical trial. By ensuring that source data is accurately and contemporaneously recorded and that CRFs are completed with meticulous attention to detail, investigators can maintain the integrity of the trial data and support the reliability of the study's findings. Source data verification, confidentiality measures, and proper retention practices further ensure that the trial is conducted in compliance with regulatory requirements and ethical standards.

7.3 Essential Documents

Essential documents are the backbone of the clinical trial record, providing a comprehensive and verifiable account of how the trial was conducted, the data generated, and the safeguards put in place to protect participants. These documents serve as evidence that the trial adhered to Good Clinical Practice (GCP) guidelines, regulatory requirements, and ethical standards. The careful management, retention, and accessibility of these essential documents are critical to ensuring the credibility of the trial's findings and facilitating regulatory inspections and audits.

The **Trial Master File (TMF)** is the central repository for essential documents in a clinical trial. It contains all the documents that demonstrate the trial was conducted in compliance with the protocol, GCP, and applicable regulations. The TMF is maintained by both the sponsor and the investigator, with each party responsible for their respective documents. Sponsors are responsible for maintaining the sponsor's TMF, which includes documents related to trial management, monitoring, and safety reporting, while investigators are responsible for maintaining the investigator's TMF, which includes documents related to participant enrollment, informed consent, and source data.

Essential documents include a wide range of records, such as the trial protocol and protocol amendments, which outline the study's design, objectives, methodology, and procedures. The protocol is the foundation of the trial, and any amendments must be carefully documented to ensure that all changes to the study are approved by regulatory authorities and ethics committees. The TMF also includes ethics committee approvals and informed consent forms, which demonstrate that the trial was reviewed and approved by an independent ethics committee and that participants were fully informed of the study's risks and benefits before enrolling.

Investigator brochures and safety reports are also key components of the essential documents. The investigator brochure provides detailed information about the investigational product, including its safety profile, pharmacology, and preclinical data. Safety reports, such as adverse events and serious adverse event reports, document any safety issues that arise during the trial and demonstrate that the sponsor and investigator took appropriate actions to protect participants.

Other essential documents include monitoring reports, audit certificates, and correspondence with regulatory authorities. Monitoring reports provide a record of the site visits conducted by CRAs, detailing the findings of each visit and any corrective actions taken in response to identified issues. Audit certificates confirm that the trial was audited for compliance with GCP, and correspondence with regulatory authorities documents any interactions with health authorities, such as requests for additional information or approval of protocol amendments.

Document retention is a critical aspect of essential document management. Regulatory authorities, such as the **U.S. Food and Drug Administration (FDA)** and the **European Medicines Agency (EMA),** require that essential documents be retained for a specified period after the conclusion of the trial, typically five to fifteen years. This retention period ensures that the documents remain available for regulatory inspections, audits, or legal proceedings. Investigators and sponsors must implement secure storage practices to protect the documents from damage, loss, or unauthorized access during the retention period.

Another important consideration is the archiving of essential documents. The documents may be archived for long-term storage at the end of the retention period. Archiving practices must comply with local regulations and GCP guidelines, ensuring that the documents remain accessible for future reference if needed. For example, if a regulatory authority requests a reanalysis of the trial data or if the investigational product receives marketing approval, the essential documents may need to be retrieved from the archives to support these activities.

Essential documents are a vital component of clinical trial management, providing a comprehensive record of the study's conduct and compliance with GCP, regulatory requirements, and ethical standards. Proper management, retention, and archiving of these documents are critical to ensuring the credibility of the trial and facilitating regulatory inspections and audits. Sponsors and investigators can demonstrate the integrity of the trial and support the investigational product's journey toward regulatory approval and clinical use by maintaining accurate and complete essential documents throughout the study.

7.4 Data Privacy and Confidentiality

Safeguarding participant information is a critical component of ethical clinical trial conduct. Data privacy and confidentiality are central to maintaining trust between participants and researchers, ensuring that sensitive information is handled with care and compliance with legal and regulatory requirements. Proper data protection measures align with Good Clinical Practice (GCP) standards, preserving the integrity of clinical research.

Data privacy laws such as the General Data Protection Regulation (GDPR) in Europe and the Health Insurance Portability and Accountability Act (HIPAA) in the United States set strict guidelines for handling personal data. These laws require that participant information be collected, stored, and used only for specific, disclosed purposes and that participants provide informed consent regarding how their data will be used. Compliance with these regulations fulfills legal obligations and reflects a commitment to participant rights and ethical research practices.

Confidentiality measures are also essential to protect participant identities. Data should be anonymized or pseudonymized wherever possible to reduce the risk of identification. Identifiable information must be securely stored and accessible only to authorized personnel. Sponsors and Clinical Research Organizations (CROs) must establish policies that strictly control access to participant data, ensuring that sensitive information is handled responsibly.

Secure data storage practices further support data privacy and confidentiality. This includes using encrypted systems to store digital data, securing physical records, and employing role-based access controls to limit data access. Regular audits and security assessments help identify potential vulnerabilities, reinforcing data protection standards.

Prioritizing data privacy and confidentiality will ensure clinical researchers uphold ethical standards, comply with regulatory requirements, and build public confidence in the research process. These efforts are essential for maintaining participant trust and supporting the credibility and reliability of clinical trial data.

7.5 Electronic Data Capture (EDC) Systems

Electronic Data Capture (EDC) systems have become fundamental in modern clinical trials, enabling efficient, accurate, and compliant data management. EDC systems are digital platforms used to collect, manage, and store trial data electronically, replacing traditional paper-based methods. These systems enhance data accessibility and streamline processes, making them indispensable tools in clinical research.

The role of EDC systems in clinical trials is multifaceted. They allow for real-time data entry and instant access to trial data across multiple sites, which is crucial for multicenter studies. By facilitating quicker data access, EDC systems enable sponsors and monitors to detect issues promptly, such as protocol deviations or data discrepancies, which can then be resolved in a timely manner. EDC systems also provide a secure environment for data storage, supporting data integrity and regulatory compliance throughout the trial.

Several best practices are essential to ensure data accuracy and reliability in EDC systems. First, data validation checks should be integrated into the system to prevent entry errors. These checks flag missing data, out-of-range values, or inconsistencies, prompting users to correct them at the point of entry. Role-based access controls should also be implemented to restrict data access to authorized personnel, preserving data confidentiality and security.

Compliance with regulatory standards such as Good Clinical Practice (GCP) and 21 CFR Part 11 is critical for EDC systems. These standards require electronic records to be traceable and secure, with audit trails documenting every data entry, modification, and deletion. Regular system audits and training for users further reinforce compliance, ensuring that data is handled correctly and ethically.

Incorporating EDC systems into clinical trials offers significant benefits in data management, quality control, and regulatory adherence, ultimately enhancing the efficiency and integrity of clinical research.

This chapter has explored the importance of data handling and record management in clinical trials, focusing on data integrity, the management of source data and CRFs, and the role of essential documents. Ensuring that data is accurate, complete, and reliable is fundamental. By maintaining meticulous records of trial activities, sponsors and investigators can ensure the success of the trial and support the ethical conduct of clinical research. Proper data management is essential for safeguarding participant safety, ensuring regulatory compliance, and generating reliable findings that can advance medical knowledge and improve patient care.

Chapter Eight

Risk Management and Quality by Design

8.1 Proactive Risk Identification

In clinical trials, proactively identifying risks is crucial for safeguarding participant safety and ensuring data integrity. Proactive risk identification involves anticipating potential challenges and threats that could arise during the trial and addressing them before they affect the study's outcomes. The goal of this process is to minimize negative impacts on trial participants, data quality, and regulatory compliance. By systematically identifying and mitigating risks at the outset, clinical research teams can create a more efficient, reliable, and ethically sound trial process.

One of the most effective strategies for identifying risks in clinical trials is conducting a comprehensive risk assessment during the trial design phase. This assessment involves analyzing all aspects of the trial—from protocol development to participant recruitment to data collection and monitoring—to pinpoint areas where risks could emerge. Key risk factors include complex study designs, investigational product safety profiles, the study population's characteristics, and the investigative sites' experience level. For example, a complex trial with multiple treatment arms may pose risks related to protocol adherence, while a study involving a vulnerable population, such as pediatric or elderly participants, may carry additional safety concerns. Understanding these potential risks allows the research team to implement strategies that prevent issues from occurring or reduce their impact if they do arise.

Stakeholder involvement is a critical element in proactive risk identification. Effective risk management requires input from all parties involved in the trial, including sponsors, investigators, clinical research organizations (CROs), and regulatory authorities. Each stakeholder brings unique insights and expertise, which can help identify risks that might otherwise be overlooked. For example, investigators at the site level can provide valuable feedback on potential operational risks, such as difficulties with patient recruitment or retention, while regulatory authorities can offer guidance on compliance risks. By fostering open communication and collaboration among all stakeholders, the research team can ensure that a broad range of risks are identified and addressed early in the trial process.

Another key strategy for identifying risks is conducting root cause analysis on previous trials. By examining past studies, sponsors and investigators can identify common challenges and potential pitfalls that could also arise in the current trial. For example, if previous trials involving a similar investigational product experienced high rates of adverse events, this information can be used to adjust the current study's protocol and implement additional safety monitoring measures. Similarly, if previous trials encountered issues with data collection, such as incomplete or inconsistent CRFs, the research team can implement enhanced data management protocols to mitigate these risks in the new trial. Lessons learned from past experiences are invaluable for proactively identifying and mitigating risks.

Risk identification tools and methodologies, such as **Failure Mode and Effects Analysis (FMEA)** or **Hazard Analysis and Critical Control Points (HACCP),** are commonly used in clinical trials to systematically assess potential risks and their impact. These tools allow research teams to identify specific points in the trial process where failures or deviations are most likely to occur and develop mitigation strategies to address these vulnerabilities. For example, FMEA involves identifying potential failure modes, assessing their likelihood and severity, and implementing controls to prevent or reduce the impact of these failures. By using structured methodologies to identify risks, research teams can create a more robust risk management plan covering all trial aspects.

Once risks have been identified, developing mitigation strategies that address each specific risk is important. Mitigation strategies may include additional safety monitoring, increased training for site staff, or enhanced data validation procedures. For example, if a trial involves a high-risk population, the research team may decide to implement more frequent safety assessments or stricter inclusion/exclusion criteria to protect participants. Similarly, if a trial is at risk for high rates of protocol deviations, the team may provide additional training for site staff or implement more frequent monitoring visits to ensure protocol adherence. Addressing risks proactively will allow research teams to minimize the likelihood of problems arising and ensure the trial runs smoothly.

Proactive risk identification is essential for ensuring the success of a clinical trial. By conducting comprehensive risk assessments involving all stakeholders, learning from past experiences, and using risk assessment tools, research teams can anticipate potential issues and implement mitigation strategies to prevent them. This proactive approach protects participant safety and ensures that the trial produces high-quality, reliable data that can support regulatory approval and inform future clinical practice.

8.2 Quality by Design (QbD) Approach

The concept of **Quality by Design (QbD)** is a structured approach to clinical trial design that integrates risk management principles to ensure the delivery of high-quality outcomes. QbD involves building quality into every aspect of the trial from the very beginning rather than relying solely on corrective actions to address issues after they arise. Incorporating quality into the trial's design and execution helps QbD ensure that the study is scientifically valid, ethically sound, and capable of generating reliable data that meets regulatory requirements.

At its core, QbD is based on the idea that quality cannot be "inspected" in a trial; it must be designed and built into the process from the outset. This means that quality considerations are integrated into every stage of the trial, from protocol development to data collection and analysis. For example, during the protocol development phase, QbD principles emphasize the importance of clearly defining the trial's objectives, endpoints, and methodology to ensure that the study is designed to answer the research question in a scientifically valid way. The protocol should be structured to minimize potential biases, reduce variability, and ensure consistency in data collection across all sites. By focusing on quality during the design phase, QbD helps prevent issues such as protocol deviations, data discrepancies, or safety concerns from compromising the trial's outcomes.

Risk management is a central component of the QbD approach, as it identifies and mitigates risks that could impact trial quality. During the trial design phase, sponsors and investigators conduct a thorough risk assessment to identify potential challenges and vulnerabilities that could arise during the study. This includes assessing risks related to participant safety, data integrity, protocol adherence, and regulatory compliance. Once risks have been identified, the QbD approach involves developing targeted mitigation strategies to address each risk and ensure that the trial is conducted with the highest level of quality. For example, if a trial is expected to enroll a diverse patient population with varying levels of health literacy, the research team may develop enhanced informed consent procedures to ensure that all participants fully understand the trial's risks and benefits.

The QbD approach also emphasizes the importance of **Critical-to-Quality (CtQ)** factors, which are the key elements of the trial that have the greatest impact on its success. CtQ factors may include specific data points, participant safety measures, or operational procedures that are essential for achieving the trial's objectives. Identifying and prioritizing these CtQ factors helps the research team focus their efforts on the aspects of the trial that matter most for ensuring quality. For example, in a clinical trial evaluating a new oncology treatment, CtQ factors might include the accuracy of tumor measurement data, adherence to dosing schedules, and timely reporting of adverse events. By focusing on these critical elements, the QbD approach helps ensure that the trial produces reliable, high-quality data that can support regulatory approval.

Another key principle of QbD is the use of robust data management and monitoring systems to ensure the accuracy and integrity of the trial data. QbD emphasizes the importance of designing data collection tools, such as Case Report Forms (CRFs) and electronic data capture (EDC) systems, that are easy to use and capable of capturing data in a consistent and standardized way. For example, CRFs should be designed to minimize the potential for data entry errors by using clearly defined fields and validation checks. EDC systems should have built-in data validation features that flag discrepancies or out-of-range values in real-time, allowing site staff to correct any errors before the data is finalized. By incorporating quality into the data collection process, QbD helps ensure that the trial produces accurate, complete, and reliable data.

The QbD approach also promotes the use of adaptive trial designs, which allow for flexibility in the conduct of the trial based on interim results or evolving information. Adaptive designs can help improve trial quality by allowing the research team to make adjustments to the protocol in response to emerging data. For example, if interim results suggest that one treatment arm is significantly more effective than the others, the trial design may be adapted to focus on the most promising treatment, thereby improving the overall quality and efficiency of the study. Adaptive designs are particularly useful in complex trials or studies involving novel therapies, where the ability to make mid-trial adjustments can significantly enhance the trial's quality and success.

The QbD approach emphasizes the importance of training and education for all members of the research team. Ensuring that investigators, site staff, monitors, and data managers are properly trained in GCP guidelines, protocol requirements, and data management procedures is essential for maintaining trial quality. Training programs should be tailored to the specific needs of the trial and should include ongoing education to address any changes in the protocol or new developments in the trial. By providing comprehensive training, the QbD approach ensures that all team members have the knowledge and skills necessary to conduct the trial with the highest level of quality.

The QbD approach integrates risk management and quality principles into every stage of the clinical trial, ensuring that quality is built into the trial's design and execution from the outset. By focusing on critical-to-quality factors, robust data management systems, adaptive trial designs, and comprehensive training, QbD helps ensure that the trial produces reliable, high-quality data supporting regulatory approval and informing future clinical practice. The QbD approach not only enhances the scientific validity of the trial but also protects participant safety and ensures compliance with regulatory requirements.

8.3 Continuous Process Improvement

Continuous process improvement is a key principle in clinical trial management. It ensures that the trial evolves and improves over time based on ongoing feedback, monitoring, and lessons learned. The concept of continuous improvement is rooted in the idea that no process is perfect and that there is always room for refinement and optimization. In the context of clinical trials, continuous process improvement involves regularly evaluating the trial's conduct, identifying areas for improvement, and implementing changes to enhance trial quality, participant safety, and data integrity.

One of the primary tools for continuous improvement in clinical trials is ongoing monitoring and feedback. Regular monitoring visits, remote data reviews, and centralized monitoring activities provide real-time feedback on the trial's progress and highlight any issues or deviations that need to be addressed. For example, if monitoring activities reveal a high rate of protocol deviations at certain sites, the research team can implement corrective actions, such as additional training for site staff or enhanced oversight at those sites. Similarly, if data monitoring identifies discrepancies or missing data in CRFs, the team can take steps to improve data collection processes and ensure that the data is complete and accurate.

Continuous process improvement also involves reviewing trial-wide trends and metrics to identify broader patterns that may indicate areas for improvement. For example, the research team may analyze data on participant recruitment rates, protocol deviations, adverse event reporting, or data query resolution times across all sites to identify trends that suggest potential inefficiencies or areas of concern. If recruitment rates are lower than expected at certain sites, the team may decide to adjust the recruitment strategy or provide additional support to those sites to improve enrollment. Similarly, if certain types of protocol deviations are consistently occurring across multiple sites, the team may revise the protocol or provide additional training to address the issue.

Root cause analysis is another important tool for continuous process improvement. When issues arise during the trial—such as a protocol deviation, data discrepancy, or safety concern—it is important to conduct a thorough analysis of the root cause of the issue to determine why it occurred and how it can be prevented in the future. For example, if a site consistently fails to report adverse events within the required timeframe, a root cause analysis may reveal that the site staff were not adequately trained on the reporting requirements. In this case, the research team can implement additional training and monitoring to ensure that the issue is resolved and does not occur again.

Corrective and preventive actions (CAPA) are a key component of continuous process improvement. When issues are identified during the trial, the research team must develop and implement corrective actions to address the immediate problem, as well as preventive actions to prevent the issue from recurring. For example, if a data management system fails to capture critical data points, the team may implement a corrective action to resolve the current data discrepancy and a preventive action to ensure that the system is updated to prevent similar issues in the future. CAPA processes help ensure that the trial continues to evolve and improve over time, ultimately leading to higher-quality outcomes.

Lessons learned from previous trials are also a valuable source of information for continuous process improvement. Sponsors and investigators can identify best practices and areas for improvement that can be applied to future trials by reviewing and considering the outcomes of past studies. For example, if a previous trial experienced challenges with participant retention, the research team may decide to implement more robust retention strategies—such as increased communication with participants or more flexible visit schedules—in the current trial. Lessons learned from past trials help ensure that the research team can anticipate potential challenges and implement solutions proactively rather than reacting to problems as they arise.

Technology and innovation play a critical role in continuous process improvement. As new technologies and methodologies are developed, research teams can incorporate these innovations into their trials to improve efficiency, data quality, and participant safety. For example, the use of electronic informed consent (eConsent) systems can streamline the consent process, improve participant understanding, and ensure that consent is properly documented. Similarly, the use of wearable devices and remote monitoring technologies can enhance the collection of real-time data and reduce the burden on participants, improving overall trial quality and participant satisfaction. By staying up to date with the latest technological advancements, research teams can continuously improve the conduct of their trials.

Continuous process improvement is essential for ensuring that clinical trials evolve and improve over time. By incorporating ongoing monitoring, feedback, root cause analysis, CAPA processes, lessons learned, and technological innovations, research teams can enhance trial quality, protect participant safety, and ensure the generation of reliable, high-quality data. Continuous improvement not only supports the ethical and scientific integrity of the trial but also ensures that the study remains adaptable and responsive to changing circumstances, ultimately leading to more successful trial outcomes.

8.4 Risk Assessment Tools and Techniques

Effective risk management in clinical trials begins with thorough risk assessment, using a variety of tools and methodologies to evaluate potential risks to participants, data integrity, and trial compliance. Understanding these risks allows for the implementation of preventive measures, ensuring trial quality and safety. Key tools for risk assessment include scoring systems, checklists, and risk matrices, each tailored to identify and prioritize risks in clinical research.

Scoring systems are commonly used to assign values to potential risks based on factors such as probability, impact, and detectability. For example, a high probability and high-impact risk, such as participant safety concerns, may receive a high score, indicating the need for immediate action. By quantifying risks in this way, scoring systems allow research teams to objectively evaluate the urgency and potential consequences of each risk, helping to allocate resources effectively.

Checklists provide a structured approach to risk assessment by ensuring that all possible risks are considered across various trial areas, from participant recruitment and data collection to site management and regulatory compliance. These checklists are particularly useful for complex, multicenter trials where the likelihood of protocol deviations, data errors, or ethical issues may increase. Using a checklist ensures that no critical areas are overlooked, supporting a thorough and systematic risk assessment process.

Risk matrices are visual tools that map risks based on their probability and impact, helping teams to prioritize risk management efforts. In a typical matrix, risks are plotted on a grid, with high-probability, high-impact risks requiring more attention than low-probability, low-impact risks. This visual representation aids in strategic decision-making, focusing resources on the most significant threats to trial quality and safety.

Together, these tools and techniques allow clinical research professionals to identify, assess, and manage risks effectively, creating a proactive environment supporting clinical trials' ethical and scientific integrity.

8.5 Risk Communication and Stakeholder Engagement

Effective risk communication is essential in clinical trials to ensure that all stakeholders, including sponsors, investigators, regulatory authorities, and ethics committees, are aligned and prepared to respond to potential risks. Transparent and timely communication fosters collaboration and supports proactive decision-making, which is crucial for maintaining the integrity and safety of the trial.

One key strategy in risk communication is establishing a structured process for sharing information across teams and stakeholders. This includes regular meetings, detailed reports, and real-time updates on emerging risks. Clear documentation, such as risk management plans and risk logs, provides a central reference for all parties, outlining identified risks, their potential impact, and mitigation strategies. Maintaining such transparency helps stakeholders understand the current risk landscape, enabling them to support the trial effectively.

Stakeholder engagement is strengthened by tailoring communication to each group's role and level of involvement. For example, investigators need detailed, practical information on how to implement risk mitigation at their sites, while sponsors and regulatory authorities may require high-level summaries that address overall trial safety and compliance. All stakeholders must have relevant information in an accessible format; clinical trial teams can enhance understanding and ensure that each stakeholder is prepared to manage risks within their specific context.

Proactive updates and early warnings play a crucial role in risk communication. If a significant issue arises, promptly notifying stakeholders allows for quicker responses, minimizing potential harm to participants and preserving data integrity. This approach requires establishing predefined communication channels and protocols for escalation, ensuring rapid information flow in urgent situations.

Fostering an open feedback loop is essential to risk communication. Encouraging stakeholders to share observations, concerns, and suggestions enhances risk identification and allows the team to continuously refine risk management practices. Research teams should promote a collaborative, communicative environment to ensure that risks are managed comprehensively, supporting the trial's ethical and scientific quality.

This chapter has explored the importance of proactive risk identification, the Quality by Design (QbD) approach, and continuous process improvement in clinical trial management. By integrating risk management and quality principles into the trial design and execution and by continuously evaluating and improving trial processes, sponsors and investigators can ensure the success of the trial and the protection of participants. These strategies not only enhance the scientific validity of the trial but also help ensure that the study meets regulatory requirements and produces reliable data that can inform future clinical practice.

Chapter Nine

Investigator Brochure

9.1 Purpose and Contents

The **Investigator Brochure (IB)** is a critical document in clinical trials, providing a comprehensive summary of information about the investigational product (IP) that is being studied. Its primary function is to ensure that investigators, sponsors, and regulatory authorities are well-informed about the investigational product's characteristics, including its pharmacological properties, safety profile, and prior testing results. By compiling all relevant preclinical and clinical data, the IB helps investigators conduct the trial safely, ethically, and in compliance with regulatory guidelines.

The IB serves as an important educational resource for the investigators, providing them with the necessary scientific foundation to understand the investigational product's mechanisms of action, potential risks, and therapeutic potential. Investigators use this document to assess the appropriateness of the trial, determine the potential benefits and risks to participants, and make informed decisions regarding patient safety during the study. Without the IB, investigators would lack crucial context, which could lead to improper use of the investigational product or poor decision-making in risk management.

The contents of the Investigator Brochure are organized into several sections, each of which provides a different aspect of information about the investigational product. Typically, the IB includes a detailed description of the drug or device, including its chemical, physical, and pharmacological properties. For a drug, this might include details about its active ingredients, formulation, solubility, and mechanism of action. For a device, it may describe its components, function, and intended therapeutic use. The IB also covers relevant preclinical data, such as animal studies showing the drug's pharmacodynamics (PD) and pharmacokinetics (PK) or its toxicological profile. This information helps investigators understand how the product behaves in biological systems, providing critical insights into its potential effects in human subjects.

The clinical data section of the IB summarizes the results of any prior human trials conducted with the investigational product. This might include Phase I studies that evaluate safety and tolerability, as well as any early indications of efficacy from Phase II trials. The IB also outlines any known side effects or adverse reactions that have been observed in previous studies, helping investigators anticipate potential safety issues in their own trials. Additionally, the IB contains information on the dosage and administration of the investigational product, including recommended dosing regimens, routes of administration, and special considerations for specific populations (such as those with renal or hepatic impairment).

An important component of the IB is its risk-benefit analysis, which weighs the potential therapeutic effects of the investigational product against the possible risks to participants. This section is particularly critical for ensuring that the trial is ethical, as it helps investigators determine whether the benefits justify exposing participants to the investigational product. The risk-benefit analysis also guides the design of the trial's safety monitoring procedures, such as the frequency of adverse event reporting or the need for specific laboratory tests to monitor participants' health.

The IB also guides investigators in handling specific situations that may arise during the trial. For example, it may include recommendations on how to manage adverse events, adjust the dosage if participants experience toxicity, or proceed if participants develop certain medical conditions during the trial. This guidance helps ensure that investigators are well-prepared to respond to potential challenges and maintain participant safety throughout the study.

The IB is an indispensable document in clinical research, providing investigators with the information they need to conduct trials safely, ethically, and effectively. Its comprehensive nature ensures that all aspects of the investigational product's safety, efficacy, and scientific rationale are well-documented, supporting informed decision-making and compliance with regulatory requirements.

9.2 Safety and Efficacy Data

One of the most crucial components of the Investigator Brochure is the safety and efficacy data section, which provides a detailed account of the nonclinical and clinical studies conducted with the investigational product. This section serves as the foundation for understanding the product's potential benefits and risks, helping investigators make informed decisions about the design and conduct of the clinical trial. By summarizing preclinical and clinical findings, the IB ensures that investigators clearly understand the investigational product's safety profile and therapeutic potential.

The nonclinical safety data section of the IB presents the results of laboratory and animal studies that have been conducted to assess the pharmacological and toxicological properties of the investigational product. These studies are essential for determining whether the product is safe to test in humans and for identifying any potential risks that may need to be monitored during the trial. For example, preclinical toxicology studies may reveal organ toxicity, reproductive toxicity, or carcinogenicity, all of which are important considerations when designing a trial involving human participants. The IB will typically include data on acute and chronic toxicity, as well as results from studies evaluating the product's impact on specific organ systems, such as the cardiovascular, renal, or hepatic systems. Understanding the investigational product's toxicological profile is essential for anticipating potential adverse events and implementing appropriate safety monitoring procedures during the trial.

The IB also includes pharmacokinetic (PK) and pharmacodynamic (PD) data, which describe how the investigational product is absorbed, distributed, metabolized, and excreted by the body, as well as how it interacts with biological targets to produce its therapeutic effects. PK data, such as the drug's half-life, bioavailability, and clearance rates, help investigators understand how long the drug remains in the body and how frequently it needs to be administered to maintain therapeutic levels. PD data, on the other hand, provide insights into the product's mechanism of action, target engagement, and dose-response relationships. Together, PK and PD data help inform dosing strategies, optimize therapeutic efficacy, and minimize the risk of adverse effects.

The clinical safety and efficacy data section of the IB summarizes the findings from any previous human studies conducted with the investigational product. This typically includes data from Phase I studies, designed to assess the product's safety, tolerability, and pharmacokinetics in healthy volunteers or in patients with the target condition. Phase I studies provide critical information on the product's safety profile, including any adverse events (AEs) or serious adverse events (SAEs) that occurred during the study. The IB also includes data from Phase II trials, which focus on assessing the product's efficacy in a larger patient population and provide early evidence of its therapeutic potential. These trials often explore different doses or regimens of the product to determine the optimal dose for future studies.

The adverse event profile of the investigational product is a key aspect of the IB's safety data. Before administering the product to trial participants, investigators must be fully aware of any known side effects or safety concerns. The IB provides detailed information on the types, severity, and frequency of adverse events observed in nonclinical and clinical studies, as well as guidance on managing these events during the trial. For example, the IB may include recommendations on dose adjustments or discontinuation criteria in the event of severe toxicity. By providing this information, the IB helps investigators anticipate potential safety issues and implement appropriate monitoring procedures to protect participants.

The efficacy data section of the IB highlights any early signs of the investigational product's therapeutic benefits based on preclinical models or Phase II trials. While early efficacy data is often limited, it can provide valuable insights into the product's potential to treat the target condition and help justify further clinical investigation. For example, if a Phase II trial demonstrated a significant reduction in tumor size or an improvement in disease symptoms, this data would support the decision to proceed with larger Phase III trials to confirm the product's efficacy in a broader patient population.

The safety and efficacy data presented in the Investigator Brochure are essential for guiding the safe and effective use of the investigational product in clinical trials. By providing a detailed account of the product's nonclinical and clinical findings, the IB helps investigators assess the product's risk-benefit profile and make informed decisions about trial design, participant safety, and therapeutic potential.

9.3 Updates and Maintenance

The Investigator Brochure (IB) is not a static document. It requires regular updates and maintenance to reflect new information that may arise during the clinical trial or from ongoing nonclinical and clinical studies. Keeping the IB up to date is crucial for ensuring that investigators have access to the most current information about the investigational product, particularly with regard to safety and efficacy data. Regular updates help protect trial participants by ensuring that any emerging risks are communicated promptly and that investigators can adjust their safety monitoring procedures accordingly.

The need for regular updates to the IB typically arises from several sources. First, as clinical trials progress and new data are generated, the sponsor must evaluate whether this information has implications for the safety or efficacy of the investigational product. For example, if a Phase II trial reveals a higher-than-expected rate of serious adverse events (SAEs) or identifies a new safety signal, this information must be included in an updated version of the IB. Similarly, if new clinical data demonstrates a significant therapeutic benefit at a particular dose, this information should be communicated to investigators to ensure that the trial is optimized for efficacy. These updates are particularly important for trials that are ongoing or for new trials that are about to start, as they allow investigators to make informed decisions based on the most recent data.

Updates to the IB may also be required if regulatory authorities request additional information or impose new safety requirements. For example, if a regulatory agency issues a safety warning related to the investigational product, the sponsor must update the IB to reflect this new information and provide guidance to investigators on how to manage the associated risks. Failure to update the IB in a timely manner could result in regulatory noncompliance, trial delays, or even termination of the study if participant safety is compromised.

The process of updating the IB typically involves a systematic review of new data, including results from ongoing nonclinical and clinical studies, safety reports, and any other relevant information that has emerged since the last version of the IB was issued. The sponsor is responsible for compiling this information, assessing its impact on the investigational product's safety and efficacy profile, and determining whether updates to the IB are warranted. Once the updates are made, the revised IB is reviewed by the sponsor's clinical and regulatory teams to ensure that it meets all relevant regulatory requirements and provides accurate, up-to-date information to investigators.

Once the revised IB is finalized, it must be distributed to all investigators participating in the clinical trial. Investigators are responsible for reviewing the updated IB and incorporating the new information into their trial procedures. This may involve updating informed consent forms, adjusting safety monitoring protocols, or modifying dosing regimens based on the new data. Investigators must also ensure that their site staff is informed of any changes and that they are properly trained on any new procedures that may be required. For example, if the updated IB identifies a new safety signal related to liver toxicity, the investigator may need to implement additional liver function tests or modify the frequency of safety assessments for participants.

The sponsor must also notify regulatory authorities and ethics committees of the changes. Regulatory authorities may require the sponsor to submit the updated IB for review and approval, particularly if the changes have significant implications for participant safety or trial conduct. Ethics committees must also review the updated IB to ensure that the trial remains ethically sound in light of the new information. This process ensures that all stakeholders know the changes and that the trial meets regulatory and ethical standards.

The need for regular updates to the IB highlights the importance of ongoing safety surveillance during clinical trials. As new data emerges, the sponsor must continuously assess the risk-benefit profile of the investigational product and ensure that any changes are communicated to investigators in a timely manner. This process protects participant safety and ensures that the trial remains scientifically valid and complies with regulatory requirements.

The IB must be regularly updated and maintained to reflect new information about the investigational product's safety and efficacy. By providing investigators with the most current data, these updates ensure that trials are conducted safely and ethically and that participant safety is protected throughout the study. Regular updates also help ensure compliance with regulatory requirements and facilitate the ongoing success of the clinical trial.

9.4 Regulatory Requirements and Compliance

The Investigator Brochure (IB) is a vital document in clinical trials, providing comprehensive information about the investigational product's safety and efficacy profile. It must adhere to international and country-specific regulatory requirements to ensure this document supports ethical and compliant trial conduct. Compliance with these regulations, including ICH GCP standards, is essential for the protection of trial participants and the reliability of trial outcomes.

ICH GCP guidelines provide the framework for creating and updating the IB. According to these guidelines, the IB should contain all preclinical and clinical data relevant to the investigational product, enabling investigators to understand potential risks, benefits, and necessary precautions. The ICH GCP guidelines specify that the IB be clear, concise, and updated as new data emerges, ensuring that investigators have access to the most current information to make informed decisions during the trial.

In addition to ICH GCP standards, country-specific regulations may impose additional requirements for the IB. For instance, some regulatory bodies, such as the U.S. Food and Drug Administration (FDA) or the European Medicines Agency (EMA), may require specific formatting, additional sections, or distinct content focuses, such as detailed risk information for vulnerable populations. Sponsors must be aware of these country-specific mandates to avoid regulatory setbacks and ensure that the IB meets all legal requirements.

Regular updates and periodic reviews are also essential for maintaining compliance. As new data from ongoing or completed studies becomes available, the IB must be promptly revised to reflect updated safety and efficacy information. This ongoing commitment to accuracy helps ensure the document remains a reliable resource for investigators, supporting participant safety and study validity.

Sponsors and research teams must adhere to ICH GCP guidelines and relevant national regulations to uphold the ethical and scientific rigor essential in clinical trials, reinforcing the credibility and trustworthiness of the research.

9.5 Distribution and Access

Effective distribution and access to the Investigator Brochure (IB) are crucial for ensuring that investigators and relevant team members are well-informed about the investigational product's safety and efficacy profile. Timely access to the most current version of the IB helps safeguard participant safety, supports protocol compliance, and enhances data reliability throughout the trial.

Best practices for IB distribution begin with establishing a systematic process for disseminating the document to all study sites. Sponsors or Clinical Research Organizations (CROs) are responsible for ensuring that each site receives the IB before study initiation and that any subsequent updates are distributed as soon as they become available. Many research teams use secure electronic platforms to distribute the IB, allowing immediate access and reducing delays associated with physical delivery. In addition, electronic distribution allows tracking of document access and acknowledgment, ensuring that all necessary parties have received and reviewed the IB.

Ensuring timely access to updates is essential, particularly when new safety data becomes available. Sponsors should implement a protocol for notifying sites of IB updates, which may include alerts via email or system notifications. Investigators must acknowledge receipt of the updated IB, confirming that they are aware of any new information that could impact participant safety or trial conduct. This acknowledgment process reinforces compliance and ensures that investigators remain informed.

Controlled access is another critical element in managing IB distribution. Access should be restricted to authorized personnel, such as investigators, sub-investigators, and other key study team members, to maintain confidentiality and data security. Role-based access controls, often available through electronic platforms, ensure that only relevant individuals can view the IB, protecting the document's sensitive information.

By implementing structured distribution processes, secure access controls, and timely updates, sponsors and CROs can ensure that the IB remains an effective resource for investigators, supporting both regulatory compliance and the ethical conduct of clinical research.

This chapter has explored the critical role of the Investigator Brochure in clinical trials, focusing on its purpose and contents, the communication of safety and efficacy data, and the importance of regular updates and maintenance. The IB is an essential document that provides investigators with the information they need to conduct trials safely, effectively, and in compliance with regulatory requirements. By ensuring that the IB is kept up to date and reflects the most current data, sponsors and investigators can work together to protect participants and ensure the success of the trial.

Chapter Ten

Clinical Trial Protocol and Protocol Amendments

10.1 Key Components of the Clinical Trial Protocol

The clinical trial protocol is the cornerstone of any clinical study, serving as a comprehensive document that outlines the trial's purpose, methodology, and procedures. It acts as a detailed blueprint that guides the execution of the trial, ensuring that all stakeholders, sponsors, investigators, monitors, and regulatory authorities are aligned on how the study will be conducted. A well-constructed protocol is crucial not only for achieving the study's scientific objectives but also for safeguarding participant safety and ensuring compliance with regulatory standards.

One of the first and most important components of a clinical trial protocol is the objectives of the study. These objectives are typically divided into two categories: primary and secondary objectives. The primary objective focuses on the main question the trial seeks to answer, often related to the efficacy or safety of the investigational product. For instance, in a Phase III trial evaluating a new drug for cancer treatment, the primary objective might be to determine whether the drug improves overall survival compared to a standard treatment. On the other hand, secondary objectives explore additional questions, such as evaluating the drug's impact on quality of life or its effect on specific biomarkers. Clearly defining these objectives ensures that the study remains focused on answering the most critical scientific questions.

Closely tied to the objectives are the endpoints, which are the measurable outcomes used to assess whether the study has met its objectives. Like objectives, endpoints are typically categorized as primary and secondary endpoints. Primary endpoints correspond to the primary objective of the study and are the main criteria for determining the trial's success. For example, in a cardiovascular study, the primary endpoint might be the reduction of major adverse cardiac events (MACE), while secondary endpoints could include changes in cholesterol levels or blood pressure. Endpoints must be clearly defined, measurable, and clinically relevant to ensure that the trial produces meaningful and interpretable data.

The study design section of the protocol is another critical component that outlines how the trial will be conducted to achieve the objectives and measure the endpoints. The study design details whether the trial will be randomized, blinded, placebo-controlled, or open-label, as well as specifying the phase of the trial (e.g., Phase I, II, or III). **Randomized Controlled Trials (RCTs)** are often considered the gold standard for evaluating the efficacy of new interventions because they minimize bias by randomly assigning participants to treatment or control groups. In contrast, open-label studies, where both the participants and investigators know which treatment is being administered, may be more appropriate in certain situations, such as dose-finding studies or observational trials.

The protocol also outlines the participant selection criteria, including inclusion and exclusion criteria that define which individuals are eligible to participate in the trial. Inclusion criteria typically specify the demographic characteristics, disease condition, and stage of illness required for entry into the study, while exclusion criteria identify factors that would disqualify an individual from participation, such as a history of certain medical conditions or the use of contraindicated medications. These criteria help ensure that the trial enrolls an appropriate and homogeneous population, reducing variability in the data and increasing the likelihood of detecting a true treatment effect.

Another essential element of the clinical trial protocol is the description of study interventions, which details the investigational product(s), dosages, and schedules for administration. In drug trials, this section describes the formulation of the investigational drug, how it will be administered (e.g., orally, intravenously), the dosing regimen (e.g., daily, weekly), and any special procedures for handling the drug. In device trials, the protocol describes the design and function of the device, how it will be used, and any required surgical or procedural steps. This section also includes details on the comparator (e.g., placebo, active control) if the trial involves a comparison between different treatments.

The statistical analysis plan is another key component of the protocol that describes how the data will be analyzed to answer the trial's objectives. This section includes information on sample size calculations, statistical methods for analyzing the primary and secondary endpoints, and plans for handling missing data or protocol deviations. A well-defined statistical analysis plan is crucial for ensuring that the trial's results are scientifically valid and can withstand regulatory scrutiny.

Safety monitoring procedures are also a vital part of the protocol, outlining how adverse events (AEs) and serious adverse events (SAEs) will be reported, documented, and reviewed throughout the trial. This section ensures that participant safety is prioritized and that any risks associated with the investigational product are closely monitored. Additionally, the protocol may describe the role of a Data Safety Monitoring Board (DSMB), which is an independent group of experts responsible for overseeing the safety of participants and reviewing interim data to determine whether the trial should continue, be modified, or be stopped early due to safety concerns or overwhelming efficacy.

The clinical trial protocol is a detailed document that outlines every aspect of the study's conduct, from its objectives and endpoints to the study design, participant selection, and safety monitoring procedures. A well-developed protocol ensures that the trial is conducted in a scientifically rigorous and ethically sound manner, providing a clear roadmap for all stakeholders involved in the study.

10.2 Protocol Amendments and Approvals

Clinical trials are dynamic in nature, and it is common for unforeseen circumstances or new information to necessitate changes to the original study protocol. These changes, known as protocol amendments, are often required to address issues such as evolving safety data, recruitment challenges, or the need for additional study procedures. Protocol amendments are essential to maintaining a trial's integrity while ensuring participant safety and compliance with regulatory requirements. However, the process for submitting and obtaining approval for protocol amendments is highly regulated to ensure that any changes are scientifically justified and ethically sound.

One of the main reasons for submitting a protocol amendment is the emergence of new safety data. For example, during the course of a trial, investigators may identify previously unknown adverse effects of the investigational product that warrant changes to the protocol. In such cases, the sponsor may need to update the safety monitoring procedures, modify the dosing regimen, or revise the inclusion and exclusion criteria to reduce the risk of harm to participants. Amendments related to safety are particularly urgent and must be submitted promptly to regulatory authorities and Institutional Review Boards (IRBs) or Independent Ethics Committees (IECs) for review.

Another common reason for protocol amendments is the need to address recruitment challenges. If the trial is not enrolling participants at the expected rate, the sponsor may decide to broaden the inclusion criteria or expand the trial to additional sites in order to meet the required sample size. Such amendments help ensure that the trial can be completed in a timely manner while still adhering to the original scientific objectives. In some cases, amendments may also involve administrative changes, such as updating the list of investigators or extending the study timeline.

Once a protocol amendment is deemed necessary, the sponsor must prepare a detailed amendment submission, which outlines the proposed changes and provides a rationale for why the changes are needed. The amendment must specify how the modifications will affect the study's objectives, design, participant population, and safety monitoring procedures. This submission is then reviewed by both regulatory authorities and the

IRB/IEC, which assess whether the proposed changes are scientifically justified and whether they pose any additional risks to participants.

Regulatory authorities, such as the U.S. Food and Drug Administration (FDA) or the European Medicines Agency (EMA), play a critical role in reviewing and approving protocol amendments. Regulatory authorities evaluate whether the proposed changes align with GCP guidelines and ensure that the trial continues to meet ethical and scientific standards. Depending on the nature of the amendment, regulatory authorities may request additional information or clarification from the sponsor before granting approval. For example, if an amendment involves changing the primary endpoint of the trial, the regulatory authority may require a detailed explanation of how the change will impact the statistical analysis and the overall interpretation of the trial results.

IRBs/IECs are responsible for reviewing protocol amendments as well to ensure that participant safety and rights are protected. The IRB/IEC evaluates whether the proposed changes alter the risk-benefit profile of the trial and whether participants need to be re-consented based on the new information. For example, if an amendment introduces new safety concerns or changes the way the investigational product is administered, participants must be informed of these changes and provided with the opportunity to re-consent to their continued participation in the trial. The IRB/IEC must also ensure that the amendment does not compromise the ethical integrity of the study and that the trial continues to comply with local and international ethical standards.

The process of obtaining approval for protocol amendments can be time-consuming and complex, particularly if the changes involve significant modifications to the study design or participant safety measures.

Sponsors must ensure that they provide all necessary documentation to regulatory authorities and IRBs/IECs and that they respond promptly to any requests for additional information. Failure to obtain timely approval for a protocol amendment can result in delays to the trial or, in some cases, suspension of the study if the changes are critical to participant safety.

Once the protocol amendment is approved, the sponsor must ensure that the revised protocol is communicated to all investigators and study personnel involved in the trial. Investigators must be fully informed of the changes and provided with updated versions of the protocol, informed consent forms, and any other relevant study documents. Investigators are responsible for implementing the changes at their sites and ensuring that participants are re-consented if necessary. Sponsors may also provide additional training to site staff to ensure that they are aware of the new procedures and can carry them out effectively.

Protocol amendments are an essential part of managing a clinical trial, allowing the study to adapt to new information or unforeseen challenges. Submitting and obtaining approval for amendments involves careful coordination between the sponsor, regulatory authorities, and IRBs/IECs to ensure that the changes are scientifically justified and ethically sound. By following a rigorous process for amending the protocol, sponsors can ensure that the trial remains compliant with regulatory requirements and continues to protect participant safety.

10.3 Managing Protocol Deviations

In the course of conducting a clinical trial, it is not uncommon for deviations from the approved protocol to occur. Protocol deviations refer to any instance in which the trial is not conducted in strict accordance with the protocol's requirements. These deviations can vary in severity, ranging from minor administrative oversights to more significant issues that could impact participant safety or data integrity. Managing protocol deviations effectively is critical for maintaining the integrity of the trial and ensuring compliance with GCP guidelines and regulatory requirements.

Minor deviations are typically administrative in nature and have little impact on the overall conduct of the trial. For example, a minor deviation might involve a participant missing a scheduled study visit by a day or receiving a laboratory test outside of the specified time window. While these deviations do not typically pose a risk to participant safety or data quality, they must still be documented and reported according to the sponsor's procedures. Investigators are responsible for documenting minor deviations in the trial records, including an explanation of the deviation and any corrective actions taken to prevent it from recurring. This documentation is important for ensuring transparency and accountability in the trial's conduct.

Major deviations, on the other hand, are more serious and may have a significant impact on the trial's outcomes or participant safety. Examples of major deviations include administering the wrong dose of the investigational product, enrolling a participant who does not meet the inclusion criteria, or failing to report a serious adverse event within the required timeframe. Major deviations must be reported to both the sponsor and regulatory authorities promptly, as they could compromise the integrity of the trial data or pose a risk to participants. In some cases, major deviations may require corrective actions, such as re-training site staff, modifying study procedures, or even withdrawing participants from the trial if their safety is at risk.

The first step in managing a protocol deviation is to identify the deviation as soon as it occurs. Investigators and site staff must be vigilant in monitoring the conduct of the trial to ensure that any deviations are detected early and reported promptly. Once a deviation is identified, the investigator must assess its severity and impact on the trial. This assessment involves determining whether the deviation affects participant safety, the scientific validity of the trial, or regulatory compliance. For example, if a participant receives a dose of the investigational product that is higher than the protocol-specified dose, the investigator must assess whether this poses a risk to the participant's health and whether the deviation could affect the study's overall findings.

After the deviation has been assessed, the investigator must take corrective and preventive actions (CAPA) to address the deviation and prevent it from recurring. Corrective actions may involve providing additional safety monitoring for the participant affected by the deviation or adjusting the trial procedures to prevent similar deviations in the future. For example, if a deviation occurs because a participant missed a scheduled study visit, the site may implement a reminder system to ensure that participants are reminded of their appointments in advance. Preventive actions are designed to address the root cause of the deviation and ensure that it does not happen again. CAPA is a key component of managing protocol deviations, as it helps ensure that the trial continues to be conducted in compliance with GCP and regulatory requirements.

Documentation and reporting of protocol deviations are critical for maintaining the trial's integrity and ensuring regulatory compliance. Investigators must document all deviations, regardless of their severity, in the trial's records, including a description of the deviation, the reasons for its occurrence, and the corrective and preventive actions taken. Major deviations must be reported to the sponsor and regulatory authorities, and in some cases, the sponsor may be required to submit a formal deviation report to regulatory agencies. This reporting process ensures that regulatory authorities are aware of any deviations that could impact participant safety or data integrity and allows them to take appropriate actions if necessary.

Investigators must also communicate protocol deviations to the trial's **Data Safety Monitoring Board (DSMB)** and, in some cases, to the IRB/IEC. The DSMB is responsible for reviewing deviations that could affect participant safety or the validity of the trial data and may recommend changes to the protocol or additional safety monitoring procedures in response to significant deviations. The IRB/IEC may also need to review major deviations to ensure that the trial continues to meet ethical standards and that participants' rights and welfare are protected.

Managing protocol deviations is a pivotal aspect of clinical trial oversight. Promptly identifying, documenting, and reporting deviations helps investigators ensure the trial complies with GCP guidelines and regulatory requirements. Implementing corrective and preventive actions helps prevent future deviations and ensures that the trial continues to be scientifically valid and ethically sound. Proper management of protocol deviations is critical for maintaining the trial's integrity and protecting participants' safety.

10.4 Protocol Feasibility Assessment

Assessing the feasibility of a clinical trial protocol is a crucial step in ensuring that the study can be successfully implemented across multiple sites while meeting operational, ethical, and scientific standards. A well-designed feasibility assessment helps to identify potential challenges in protocol execution, reducing the risk of delays, deviations, or data quality issues that could compromise the study's outcomes.

The primary objective of a feasibility assessment is to determine if the protocol is realistically achievable within the clinical environment. This involves evaluating various factors, including participant recruitment targets, the availability of necessary resources, and the workload for site personnel. For example, a protocol with overly complex procedures or a high frequency of participant visits may be difficult for sites to implement, particularly in busy or resource-limited settings. By identifying these challenges early, sponsors and investigators can adjust the protocol or provide additional resources to ensure that the study can be conducted as planned.

Alignment with clinical operations is another critical component of feasibility assessment. The protocol must fit seamlessly within each site's operational capabilities, from staffing and training to equipment and facilities. Feasibility assessments often involve direct input from investigators and site personnel, who can provide valuable insights into site-specific constraints or requirements. This collaborative approach helps to ensure that the protocol is compatible with the practical realities of site operations.

Conducting a thorough feasibility assessment benefits the overall study by reducing the likelihood of amendments or protocol deviations, which can disrupt study timelines and introduce data variability. It also promotes participant safety, as sites are better prepared to handle the study's demands, ensuring that protocol requirements do not overburden staff or compromise care quality.

Ultimately, protocol feasibility assessments are essential for aligning scientific goals with operational practicality, supporting successful trial execution and reliable data collection across all study sites.

10.5 Documentation and Communication of Protocol Changes

Effectively managing protocol changes is essential in clinical trials to ensure that all stakeholders remain aligned and that the trial maintains compliance with regulatory standards. When a protocol modification is necessary—whether due to safety concerns, scientific insights, or operational challenges—proper documentation and clear communication are crucial to upholding the study's integrity.

Documenting protocol changes is the first step in this process. Each amendment must be meticulously recorded, detailing the rationale, specific modifications, and anticipated impact on the trial's objectives, methodology, or participant safety. These changes should be compiled in an amendment document, which becomes part of the official trial records. Accurate and thorough documentation ensures that each change is traceable, supporting regulatory compliance and enabling future reviews or audits. It also protects the study's scientific rigor, as documentation provides a clear rationale for each modification.

Clear communication of protocol changes is equally important. Stakeholders, including site staff, ethics committees, and regulatory bodies, must be informed promptly and comprehensively to ensure seamless implementation of the updated protocol. Communication with site staff should include training on any new procedures or requirements, helping to prevent errors and maintain consistency in data collection. For regulatory authorities and ethics committees, timely submissions of protocol amendments are essential, as these bodies need to review and approve changes before implementation.

Best practices for communicating protocol changes include using centralized communication platforms and standardized templates to ensure that updates are easily accessible and clearly understood. Sponsors often employ a layered approach, issuing formal amendment documents, providing training resources, and holding meetings to address any questions or concerns. This structured communication process helps align all parties, ensuring smooth transitions and continued compliance.

Clinical research teams must uphold transparency, regulatory adherence, and data integrity by prioritizing meticulous documentation and effective communication. This will ultimately support the trial's success and participant safety.

This chapter has explored the key components of the clinical trial protocol, the process for submitting and approving protocol amendments, and the management of protocol deviations. The protocol serves as the foundation for the trial's conduct, outlining the study's objectives, endpoints, and procedures, while protocol amendments allow the trial to adapt to new information or challenges. Managing protocol deviations effectively ensures that the trial remains compliant with regulatory requirements and that participant safety and data integrity are maintained throughout the study.

Chapter Eleven

Essential Records for the Conduct of a Clinical Trial

11.1 Essential Document Categories

Clinical trials generate numerous records that must be meticulously maintained to ensure compliance with regulatory standards, safeguard the data's integrity, and protect participants' rights and safety. These documents are often referred to as essential documents, and they serve as the backbone of a trial's accountability. They provide evidence that the trial was conducted per Good Clinical Practice (GCP) guidelines, regulatory requirements, and the approved protocol. Essential documents are categorized based on when they are created and used in the trial lifecycle: before, during, and after the trial.

Before the trial begins, certain documents are required to ensure that all necessary approvals have been obtained and that the trial is prepared to proceed. These documents typically include the clinical trial protocol, informed consent forms, Investigator's Brochure (IB), and regulatory bodies and ethics committees (IRBs/IECs) approvals. The clinical trial protocol is perhaps the most critical document in this phase, as it outlines the study design, objectives, endpoints, and procedures. It is accompanied by the informed consent forms, which must be reviewed and approved by an IRB/IEC to ensure they clearly explain the study's risks and benefits to potential participants. Additionally, contractual agreements, such as **Clinical Trial Agreements (CTAs)** between sponsors and investigative sites and insurance certificates to cover participants in case of injury, are also categorized as pre-trial documents.

Numerous documents are created during the trial to capture the study's progress and ensure it is conducted per the approved protocol. These include **Case Report Forms (CRFs)**, which document participant data such as medical histories, laboratory results, and treatment outcomes. CRFs are essential for tracking participant progress and ensuring data is collected consistently and accurately across all trial sites. Other essential documents during the trial phase include source documents, which are the original records of clinical observations (such as patient charts or laboratory reports), and monitoring reports, which provide evidence that the sponsor or Clinical Research Associate (CRA) has regularly reviewed the trial's progress and ensured compliance with the protocol and GCP.

The **Trial Master File (TMF)** and **Investigator Site File (ISF)** are critical repositories that house all the essential documents for the trial. The sponsor maintains the TMF and includes all documents related to trial management, regulatory submissions, and study oversight. In contrast, the ISF is maintained at each investigative site and contains site-specific documents, such as participant consent forms, source documents, and site monitoring reports. The TMF and ISF are essential for demonstrating that the trial complied with GCP and regulatory requirements. Their completeness is critical for audit and inspection readiness, as regulators rely on these files to verify the integrity of the trial.

After the trial concludes, additional documents are required to close the study and fulfill all regulatory obligations. These post-trial documents include final **Clinical Study Reports (CSRs)** summarizing the trial's results and assessing the investigational product's safety and efficacy. The CSR is a crucial document submitted to regulatory authorities for review and potential approval of the investigational product. Other post-trial documents include financial records, which detail payments made to investigators and trial participants, and closeout reports, which provide a final assessment of the trial's conduct and compliance with the protocol.

Essential documents are categorized based on their role before, during, and after the trial. They include protocols, informed consent forms, CRFs, monitoring reports, and other critical records that provide a complete and transparent account of the trial's conduct. Maintaining these documents in the TMF and ISF is critical for ensuring compliance with GCP guidelines, protecting participants, and supporting regulatory submissions.

11.2 Document Retention and Archiving

Once a clinical trial has concluded, it is essential to ensure that all trial-related documents are retained and archived according to regulatory requirements. Document retention is critical for enabling future audits, inspections, and regulatory reviews, and preserving the trial's data in case of post-trial analyses or safety concerns. The regulations governing document retention vary depending on the jurisdiction. All essential documents must be retained for a specified period after the trial's completion—often for several years.

In the United States, for example, the Food and Drug Administration (FDA) requires that trial documents be retained for at least two years following the approval of the investigational product or, if the product is not approved, for at least two years after the trial's termination. In the European Union, the European Medicines Agency (EMA) requires retention for a minimum of 25 years for certain types of records, while the International Council for Harmonisation (ICH) E6 (R3) guidelines specify retention periods that allow regulators and sponsors sufficient time to evaluate the data if needed. Sponsors and investigators must familiarize themselves with these retention requirements to ensure compliance and avoid potential regulatory penalties.

The retention process involves transferring all trial-related documents to a secure archiving system that ensures the integrity and accessibility of the records over time. This archiving process must be carried out to protect the confidentiality and security of the data. For example, physical records must be stored in locked, fireproof cabinets in a secure location. In contrast, electronic records must be housed in secure, password-protected systems that comply with data protection regulations such as the EU's General Data Protection Regulation (GDPR) or the Health Insurance Portability and Accountability Act (HIPAA) in the United States. Electronic archiving systems must also be validated to ensure that they maintain the integrity of the data, including the ability to track any changes made to the records through audit trails.

Another critical consideration in document retention is the accessibility of the archived documents. Even though the documents are no longer actively used, they must remain accessible to regulatory authorities, sponsors, and investigators upon request. This means that sponsors must have a system that allows for the quick retrieval of records, whether they are stored in physical or electronic form. In some cases, regulators may require access to these records long after the trial closed, specifically if there are safety concerns or questions about the data's validity.

While document retention is critical for compliance, it also is essential in evaluating the investigational product's safety and efficacy. Post-market surveillance and long-term safety monitoring may require sponsors and investigators to revisit trial data years after the product has been approved. Retaining comprehensive records allows for detailed reanalysis of the trial data, particularly if new safety signals emerge or if further research is needed to support additional regulatory submissions. For example, if an unexpected safety issue arises with an approved drug, the archived trial data can be reexamined to determine whether any early warning signs were missed during the initial review.

Sponsors must also develop clear archiving policies and procedures to ensure that documents are appropriately managed throughout the retention period. These policies should outline the roles and responsibilities of the personnel involved in document archiving, the procedures for transferring documents to the archive, and the measures in place to ensure document security and confidentiality. Sponsors must also establish a document destruction policy that specifies when and how documents should be destroyed after the required retention period has elapsed. Document destruction must be carried out in a way that ensures the complete and secure disposal of the records, such as through shredding physical documents or permanently deleting electronic records from storage systems.

The retention and archiving of essential trial documents are vital for ensuring compliance with regulatory requirements, protecting the integrity of the trial's data, and supporting post-trial analyses and safety monitoring. Sponsors and investigators must adhere to regulatory guidelines for document retention, implement secure archiving systems, and ensure that records remain accessible for future audits and inspections. Clear policies and procedures for document archiving and destruction are critical for maintaining the integrity and confidentiality of the trial data over time.

11.3 Auditing and Inspection Readiness

Clinical trials are subject to rigorous oversight by regulatory authorities to ensure that they are conducted following GCP guidelines, ethical principles, and applicable regulations. One of the primary mechanisms for ensuring compliance is through audits and inspections, which involve a thorough review of the trial's essential documents, processes, and data. Maintaining complete, accurate, and accessible records is critical for demonstrating that the trial has been conducted ethically and complies with regulatory standards. This section explores the importance of audit and inspection readiness and how sponsors and investigators can prepare for these reviews.

An audit is an independent evaluation of the trial's conduct completed by the sponsor or an external auditor. Audits are designed to assess the trial's adherence to the protocol, GCP, and regulatory requirements and to identify any deficiencies or areas for improvement. Auditors typically review a wide range of essential documents, including the protocol, CRFs, informed consent forms, monitoring reports, and source documents, to ensure that the trial's data is accurate and that participant safety has been maintained. Audits may include interviews with investigators, site staff, and participants to verify that the trial was conducted as documented.

To prepare for an audit, sponsors, and investigators must ensure that all essential documents are complete and current. This includes maintaining accurate participant data records, adverse event reporting, protocol deviations, and informed consent. Incomplete or inaccurate records can lead to findings of non-compliance, which may result in delays, additional oversight, or even the suspension of the trial. Sponsors must also ensure that all documents are appropriately filed and stored in the TMF and ISF, and that they are easily accessible for review by auditors.

An important aspect of audit readiness is ensuring the trial's monitoring and quality control procedures are well-documented. Auditors will review the sponsor's monitoring plans and reports to ensure that the trial was adequately monitored and that any issues were identified and addressed promptly. This includes verifying that source data was regularly checked for accuracy and completeness, that CRFs were completed correctly, and that any protocol deviations were reported and managed appropriately. Maintaining a clear audit trail that documents all monitoring activities and corrective actions is essential for demonstrating compliance and ensuring the credibility of the trial's data.

Clinical trials are also subject to inspections by regulatory authorities. Inspections are typically more comprehensive than audits and are conducted by government agencies like the FDA, EMA, or national regulatory bodies. Inspections may be conducted during the trial or after its completion and are designed to assess the trial's compliance with GCP, regulatory requirements, and ethical standards. Inspections are often triggered by specific concerns, such as reports of serious adverse events or significant protocol deviations, but they may also be conducted as part of routine regulatory oversight.

Preparing for a regulatory inspection requires a high level of organizational readiness. Sponsors and investigators must ensure that all essential documents are organized, complete, and readily accessible for inspector review. This includes trial-related documents and any regulatory submissions, such as **Investigational New Drug (IND)** applications or **Investigational Device Exemption (IDE)** applications, as well as correspondence with regulatory authorities. Sponsors should conduct mock inspections to identify gaps in documentation or procedures and ensure that all personnel are familiar with the inspection process.

During an inspection, regulatory authorities will typically review the trial's source documents, informed consent forms, and CRFs to verify the accuracy and integrity of the data. Inspectors will also evaluate the trial's safety monitoring procedures, including how adverse events were reported and managed and whether participant safety was adequately protected throughout the study. In cases where significant deviations or non-compliance are identified, inspectors may issue findings that require corrective actions or additional oversight. In severe cases, non-compliance may result in the suspension or termination of the trial.

A key component of inspection readiness is ensuring that study personnel are properly trained and knowledgeable about the trial's procedures and requirements. Investigators and site staff should be prepared to answer questions from inspectors about the trial's conduct, data collection methods, and participant safety measures. Sponsors should provide ongoing training to site staff to ensure they are familiar with GCP guidelines, the protocol, and any recent protocol amendments. A well-trained and knowledgeable team is essential for demonstrating that the trial was conducted per regulatory standards and that participant safety was a top priority.

Maintaining complete, accurate, and easily accessible records ensures audit and inspection readiness in clinical trials. Sponsors and investigators must be diligent in their documentation practices, ensuring that all essential documents are appropriately maintained in the TMF and ISF and that monitoring and quality control activities are well-documented. Preparing for audits and inspections requires a proactive approach, including regular internal reviews, mock inspections, and ongoing training for site staff. Sponsors can ensure that their trials comply with regulatory requirements and are ready for audits or inspections by maintaining high documentation standards and organizational readiness.

11.4 Electronic Document Management Systems (EDMS)

Electronic Document Management Systems (EDMS) have transformed clinical trial management by enabling secure, organized, and efficient handling of essential trial documents. These systems are critical in ensuring that all necessary records, from study protocols and investigator brochures to informed consent forms and monitoring reports, are stored and accessible in a centralized, digital format. By streamlining document storage and retrieval, EDMS enhances compliance with Good Clinical Practice (GCP) standards and regulatory requirements.

An EDMS offers centralized storage where all trial documents are securely managed. This centralization reduces the risk of document loss, simplifies file access across multiple sites, and provides a single, reliable source of up-to-date information. Essential documents are stored in an organized structure that enables rapid retrieval, supports efficient audits and inspections, and ensures that documents are readily available whenever needed.

Security and access control are fundamental components of EDMS, as clinical trial documents often contain sensitive information. EDMS platforms typically incorporate encryption, role-based access controls, and audit trails to safeguard data integrity and confidentiality. Role-based access allows different user levels, such as monitors, investigators, and sponsors, to access only the information necessary for their role, minimizing the risk of unauthorized access or data breaches. Audit trails further support transparency by tracking all document interactions, such as viewing, editing, or sharing, and creating a detailed log for compliance verification.

EDMS enables version control and real-time document tracking. Version control ensures that all stakeholders work with the latest approved versions of documents, preventing errors arising from outdated information. Real-time tracking and alerts notify users of document updates or required actions, enhancing team coordination and compliance.

An EDMS supports ethical and regulatory requirements for clinical trials, reinforcing data integrity, accessibility, and audit readiness across the trial lifecycle by securely managing, storing, and tracking essential documents.

11.5 Document Version Control and Updates

Document version control is essential in clinical trials to ensure all stakeholders work with the most current and approved versions of critical documents. Proper version control minimizes confusion, reduces the risk of protocol deviations, and supports regulatory compliance by providing a clear, traceable history of document updates.

Best practices for managing document versions begin with implementing a standardized version control system. This system should assign a unique version number to each iteration of a document, typically using a numbering format (e.g., Version 1.0, 1.1, 2.0) that indicates major and minor updates. Major updates, such as protocol amendments, warrant a full version change, while minor revisions, like corrections or clarifications, may be tracked as incremental updates. Maintaining a consistent version numbering system allows stakeholders to easily identify the latest approved document.

An effective version control system should also log each update with details on the nature of the change, the date, and the individual responsible. This documentation provides a comprehensive history of document modifications, which is essential for audit trails and regulatory inspections. A dedicated version history section within the document or in the Electronic Document Management System (EDMS) helps maintain this information in a centralized location.

Ensuring accessibility to the most recent versions is critical. EDMS platforms often feature real-time document tracking and automated alerts, notifying stakeholders when a new version is available. This functionality prevents stakeholders from inadvertently using outdated documents, supporting compliance and consistency across the trial.

To further enhance communication, sponsors and Clinical Research Organizations (CROs) should conduct training or send notifications upon releasing a new document version, especially if the update includes significant changes impacting trial conduct.

Following these best practices can ensure clinical trial teams maintain precise version control, enhance data integrity, and ensure that all stakeholders have access to accurate and up-to-date documentation.

This chapter explored the essential records required for conducting a clinical trial, the importance of document retention and archiving, and the need for audit and inspection readiness. Essential documents are the foundation of clinical trial accountability, providing a clear and transparent record of the trial's conduct and compliance with GCP guidelines and regulatory standards. Proper document management, retention, and preparation for audits and inspections are critical for ensuring trial success and protecting participants' rights and safety.

Chapter Twelve

Annex 2 – GCP Considerations for Evolving Clinical Trial Designs

12.1 Annex 2 of the ICH GCP E6(R3)

Annex 2 of the ICH GCP E6(R3) guideline expands upon the principles outlined in Annex 1 by addressing GCP considerations relevant to emerging clinical trial designs and data sources. As clinical research evolves to include decentralized elements, pragmatic elements, and real-world data (RWD), Annex 2 provides guidance on applying GCP to safeguard participant rights, safety, and well-being while ensuring trial reliability. Although not exhaustive, Annex 2 outlines critical considerations that apply across various operational approaches, with relevance shaped by local regulatory requirements. It emphasizes flexibility and quality by design (QbD) as central to ensuring trials remain scientifically valid and ethically sound.

Annex 2 of the ICH GCP E6(R3) guideline builds upon the foundational principles outlined in Annex 1, offering a focused discussion on Good Clinical Practice (GCP) considerations for emerging trial designs and data sources. With the clinical research landscape increasingly incorporating innovative approaches such as decentralized trials, pragmatic trials, and real-world data (RWD), Annex 2 provides essential guidance on adapting GCP principles to these novel methodologies. The annex underscores the importance of maintaining participant rights, safety, and well-being while ensuring clinical trial data's reliability and validity.

One of the key aspects of Annex 2 is its acknowledgment of the diversity in trial designs and data sources. It recognizes that traditional GCP frameworks may not directly apply to these emerging approaches and that tailored strategies may be necessary. For example, decentralized trials—characterized by remote monitoring, digital data collection, and direct-to-patient investigational product delivery—require careful consideration of data integrity, participant confidentiality, and effective communication between trial stakeholders. Similarly, pragmatic trials aiming to evaluate interventions under routine clinical conditions must balance scientific rigor with practical applicability to ensure meaningful results.

Annex 2 emphasizes that while the specifics of implementation may vary, the core principles of GCP remain unchanged. These principles include prioritizing participant safety, maintaining data integrity, and ensuring that trials are ethically conducted. To achieve these goals, the annex highlights the need for adaptability and a proactive approach to trial design and execution. This flexibility allows sponsors and investigators to address challenges specific to innovative trial types while upholding the overarching goals of GCP.

Annex 2 acknowledges the variability in local regulatory requirements and encourages stakeholders to consider these when applying GCP principles. While the annex provides a global framework, it recognizes that implementation must be tailored to align with specific regional regulations and cultural contexts. This emphasis on contextual relevance reinforces the guideline's flexible yet robust standards for clinical research.

Annex 2 of the ICH GCP E6(R3) guideline offers critical guidance on applying GCP principles to innovative trial designs and data sources. By emphasizing flexibility, Quality by Design, and participant-centric approaches, it ensures that clinical research continues to evolve responsibly while maintaining the highest ethical and scientific integrity standards.

12.2 Decentralized Elements in Clinical Trials

Decentralized trial elements involve conducting trial-related activities outside the traditional investigator site, leveraging innovative approaches to improve accessibility and participant experience. Common examples include home visits by healthcare professionals for assessments or sample collection, remote consultations using telehealth platforms, and utilizing **Digital Health Technologies (DHTs)** like wearable devices or mobile applications to capture real-time health data. These strategies offer significant advantages, such as reducing the logistical and time burdens on participants, increasing inclusivity by reaching underrepresented populations, and enhancing participant retention by minimizing disruptions to daily life.

Annex 2 underscores the necessity of tailored risk management plans to address these complexities. Such plans should identify potential risks unique to decentralized approaches and outline mitigation strategies, such as robust training programs for participants and trial staff to ensure the correct use of digital tools and adherence to trial protocols. Clear communication channels between sponsors, investigators, participants, and IRBs/IECs are also essential for addressing concerns, resolving issues, and ensuring that ethical and regulatory requirements are consistently met.

However, implementing decentralized trial elements introduces unique challenges that require careful attention to maintain compliance with Good Clinical Practice (GCP). Ensuring the security and integrity of remotely collected data is paramount, as data transmitted through digital platforms may be vulnerable to breaches or unauthorized access. Strict encryption protocols, secure data transfer mechanisms, and adherence to data protection regulations such as GDPR or HIPAA are critical to safeguarding participant information. Additionally, maintaining the quality and reliability of data collected through a DHT requires thorough validation of these devices and systems to confirm their accuracy and consistency in diverse real-world conditions.

Annex 2 emphasizes collaboration and proactive planning to ensure that decentralized trial elements enhance accessibility and inclusivity while maintaining the highest standards of participant safety, data integrity, and trial reliability.

12.3 Pragmatic Elements in Clinical Trials

Pragmatic trials are designed to integrate elements of routine clinical practice into the research process, bridging the gap between controlled trial environments and real-world healthcare settings. These trials often employ simplified protocols, reduced participant burdens, and streamlined data collection methods to reflect the realities of everyday clinical care. Doing so enhances the generalizability and applicability of trial findings, making the results more relevant for healthcare decision-making and policy development. However, implementing pragmatic trial designs requires meticulous planning to ensure adherence to Good Clinical Practice (GCP) principles while preserving their practical advantages.

Annex 2 highlights the importance of balancing simplicity with scientific rigor in pragmatic trials. While the reduced complexity of these trials improves feasibility and participant engagement, it must not compromise the quality or integrity of the data collected. Careful attention must be paid to maintaining robust monitoring procedures, validating data sources, and accurately assessing critical endpoints. Additionally, sponsors and investigators must provide comprehensive training for all stakeholders to familiarize them with the pragmatic aspects of the trial while ensuring compliance with the protocol and GCP requirements.

Ethical oversight is paramount in pragmatic trials. IRBs/IECs are critical in evaluating whether the trial's design safeguards participant rights, safety, and welfare while achieving its intended scientific objectives. This collaborative approach ensures that pragmatic trials maintain the highest ethical and scientific standards.

12.4 Incorporating Real-World Data (RWD) in Clinical Trials

Real-World Data (RWD) encompasses information collected outside the controlled environment of traditional clinical trials, including electronic health records (EHRs), patient registries, insurance claims data, and data from wearable devices or health apps. Integrating RWD into clinical trials offers significant potential to enhance research by providing insights into real-world patient outcomes, supporting endpoint determination, serving as external control data, or informing post-market safety and efficacy studies. This approach can also reduce trial time and cost while increasing findings' applicability to broader patient populations.

However, using RWD introduces challenges, particularly in ensuring the data's accuracy, consistency, and relevance to the trial objectives. Variability in data quality, incomplete records, and potential biases inherent in real-world sources can compromise the reliability of trial outcomes if not addressed. Annex 2 emphasizes the need for robust data validation procedures to verify the integrity and completeness of RWD, ensuring it meets the same rigorous standards as data collected within the trial.

Clear data governance frameworks are critical for managing RWD's collection, storage, and use. These frameworks must comply with privacy regulations such as GDPR or HIPAA to safeguard participant confidentiality. Investigators must align RWD with trial objectives to ensure it complements primary data collection without introducing conflicting information. Sponsors are encouraged to implement Quality by Design (QbD) principles to evaluate the suitability of RWD sources and mitigate risks associated with using secondary data. By addressing these considerations, RWD can enhance the value and efficiency of clinical trials while maintaining compliance with ethical and regulatory standards.

12.5 Quality by Design (QbD) Across All Approaches

Annex 2 emphasizes the critical role of a Quality by Design (QbD) approach in clinical trial design, operations, and data management. QbD ensures that trial methodologies and technologies are purposefully aligned with study objectives, enabling efficient, reliable, and high-quality data collection. By integrating fit-for-purpose elements into the trial design, sponsors and investigators can proactively identify and mitigate potential risks, ensuring compliance with regulatory, ethical, and scientific requirements. This approach supports the robustness and adaptability needed for modern trial methodologies, such as decentralized elements, pragmatic designs, and real-world data (RWD) integration.

The guidance in Annex 2 equips clinical research professionals with practical tools for adapting Good Clinical Practice (GCP) principles to evolving trial designs. It underscores the importance of maintaining participant safety, data reliability, and ethical integrity in increasingly complex and innovative research environments. Flexibility is a cornerstone of QbD, enabling trials to address unique challenges associated with diverse operational methods and data sources while adhering to GCP standards.

Annex 2 fosters a structured, systematic approach to ensure that even novel trial designs meet the highest regulatory and scientific standards. This balanced focus on innovation and compliance ensures that clinical trials remain participant-centric, ethically sound, and capable of producing reliable, meaningful results for healthcare advancements.

This chapter elaborates on Annex 2, which provides critical guidance for applying Good Clinical Practice (GCP) principles to innovative trial designs, including decentralized and pragmatic trials and those utilizing real-world data (RWD). By emphasizing Quality by Design (QbD), flexibility, and rigorous data governance, it ensures participant safety, ethical compliance, and data reliability across diverse and evolving clinical trial methodologies.

Chapter Thirteen

Conclusion

Summary and Final Thoughts

This book, *ICH - GCP Good Clinical Practice (GCP) E6(R3) Comprehensive Resource Guide for Clinical Research Professionals: Practical Insights and Key Updates for Clinical Study Design and Application*, has provided a thorough exploration of the ICH GCP guidelines, with a specific focus on the latest updates in E6(R3). Through practical explanations and detailed discussions, each chapter has delved into the critical aspects of clinical trial management, helping research professionals understand the standards necessary to conduct ethical, compliant, and scientifically valid studies.

In **Chapter 1**, we introduced the essence of ICH GCP, emphasizing its evolution, significance, and foundational role in global clinical research. We explored its core principles, such as safeguarding participant rights, ensuring data integrity, and maintaining ethical standards. Additionally, we highlighted the critical roles played by key stakeholders, including sponsors, investigators, Institutional Review Boards (IRBs), and regulatory authorities, who work collaboratively to uphold the integrity, reliability, and ethical conduct of clinical trials worldwide.

Chapter 2 delved into the investigator's critical responsibilities, emphasizing their role in safeguarding participant welfare, ensuring proper management and accountability of investigational products, maintaining the accuracy and integrity of trial data, and fostering effective collaboration with sponsors, monitors, and other trial partners to uphold the ethical and scientific standards of the study.

Chapter 3 highlighted the sponsor's key obligations: implementing robust quality management systems, ensuring timely safety reporting, and developing scientifically sound and ethical protocols. Additionally, it underscored the importance of selecting qualified investigators, providing them with necessary training and resources, and offering ongoing support to ensure a well-executed and compliant trial.

In **Chapter 4**, we explored the critical role of IRBs/IECs in ensuring ethical oversight of clinical trials. It detailed their responsibilities in conducting ongoing reviews of trial activities, overseeing the informed consent process to protect participant autonomy, and carefully assessing the balance between risks and benefits to safeguard participant safety and well-being.

Chapter 5 focused on adopting computerized systems in clinical trials, highlighting the necessity of system validation to ensure functionality and accuracy. It addressed critical aspects such as robust data security measures, controlled access to sensitive information, and continuous system monitoring to protect data integrity and uphold strict regulatory compliance standards.

Chapter 6 provided an in-depth look at monitoring and auditing practices, emphasizing the implementation of risk-based monitoring to focus resources on critical trial aspects. It also outlined the importance of corrective and preventive actions (CAPA) to address issues effectively and ensure trials are conducted with transparency, accountability, and adherence to high-quality standards.

Chapter 7 reviewed the critical aspects of data handling and record management, emphasizing the importance of safeguarding data privacy and using Electronic Data Capture (EDC) systems effectively. It also highlighted the necessity of maintaining comprehensive and accurate essential documents to ensure reliable trial records and regulatory compliance throughout the study.

Chapter 8 delved into risk management principles and Quality by Design (QbD), providing practical tools for proactively identifying and assessing potential risks. It emphasized effective communication strategies, continuous process improvement, and integrating QbD principles to minimize risks, enhance trial efficiency, and maintain the highest quality standards.

In **Chapter 9**, we examined the Investigator Brochure, a crucial document offering investigators comprehensive, up-to-date information about the investigational product, including its safety, efficacy, and clinical usage. The chapter highlighted the importance of ensuring compliance with regulatory requirements, maintaining accuracy, and adhering to best practices in preparing and distributing this essential resource.

Chapter 10 centered on clinical trial protocol development, covering every stage from initial feasibility assessments to the thorough documentation and management of protocol amendments. It emphasized the importance of creating adaptable and practical protocols that align with clinical operations while maintaining scientific rigor, regulatory compliance, and the overall goals of the study.

Chapter 11 outlined a comprehensive overview of the essential records required for clinical trials, detailing best practices for document retention, secure archiving, and effective management systems. It emphasized the importance of version control to ensure accuracy and highlighted these practices' critical role in maintaining audit readiness and meeting regulatory compliance standards.

Finally, **Chapter 12** discussed Annex 2 of ICH GCP E6(R3) which provides practical guidance for applying GCP principles to modern trial designs, including decentralized and pragmatic approaches and real-world data (RWD) integration. It emphasizes flexibility, Quality by Design (QbD), and collaboration to safeguard participant safety, ensure data reliability, and maintain ethical standards in evolving clinical research methodologies.

Together, these chapters provide a robust and comprehensive framework for navigating the complexities of clinical trials in alignment with ICH GCP E6(R3) guidelines. They equip clinical research professionals with the tools and knowledge needed to address the diverse challenges of modern clinical trials, from protocol development to data management and ethical oversight. By integrating these insights, professionals can strengthen their understanding of global standards, prioritize participant welfare, and uphold the integrity of trial data. This framework ensures compliance with regulatory requirements and fosters the success, ethical conduct, and scientific reliability that underpin clinical research advancements.

My parting wish is that if this guide provided valuable insights, please consider leaving a review on Amazon. Your feedback helps others discover and trust this essential resource and supports clinical research professionals worldwide in finding accurate, reliable guidance. Thank you again for reading!

About the Author

Alec Spinelli is an experienced clinical research professional who has worked in various roles in Clinical Research, including Senior CRA and Lead CRA, Clinical Site Manager, Clinical Team Lead, Clinical Trial Manager, and Project Manager. He has a strong background in Cardiology and Oncology therapeutic areas. Alec brings a wealth of expertise and extensive knowledge from his Clinical Research career that he imparts to the readers in this informative and insightful guide.

Alec holds an MBA in Business Management from Liberty University and attended the Master's Degree Program in Biomedical Engineering from Rutgers University. He also earned a Bachelor of Arts in Biology from Rutgers University, where he developed a solid foundation in the life sciences.

With over 26 years of experience in the Healthcare industry, 16 years focused on clinical research in the CRO, biotechnology, and sponsor industries, Alec has worked on clinical trials in various phases, including Phase I to Phase IV, site start-up, feasibility, pivotal IDE, and post-market studies. He has experience in clinical trial management, on-site and remote monitoring, study audits, CAPA, clinical data management, and clinical site contracts. He has extensive experience with ICG-GCP guidelines in clinical trial applications.

Alec's experience extends beyond the United States. He has worked on global clinical studies, leading cross-functional teams and collaborating with international stakeholders. He has managed clinical deliverables across multiple regions, including North America, Latin America, and Asia Pacific, demonstrating his ability to navigate diverse cultural and regulatory landscapes.

Alec has consistently demonstrated exceptional communication skills throughout his career, fostering strong relationships with investigators, study coordinators, and cross-functional teams. Alec remains proactive in expanding his knowledge of industry best practices and technological advancements. He stays informed about the latest trends in clinical research and actively participates in industry conferences, webinars, and professional organizations.

Alec Spinelli is a highly skilled and experienced Clinical Research Professional with a solid track record. With a passion for continuous learning and professional development, Alec wanted to provide this guide of ICH-GCP E6(R3) insights and updates that he complied with and uses regularly in his daily work on global clinical research trials to all clinical research professionals. He hopes you will also benefit from this comprehensive guide and successfully apply this information to your clinical research career!

www.ingramcontent.com/pod-product-compliance
Lightning Source LLC
Chambersburg PA
CBHW071029240526
45469CB00006BD/2146